PRACTICAL RECORD BOOK FOR PSYCHIATRIC/MENTAL HEALTH NURSING

Name of the Candidate : ....

Name of the Institution : ....

PRACTICAL RECORD BOOK FOR
PSYCHIATRIC/MENTAL HEALTH NURSING

Name of the Candidate: ....

Name of the Institution: ....

PRACTICAL RECORD BOOK FOR PSYCHIATRIC/MENTAL HEALTH NURSING

SECOND EDITION

Ellen Beck RN RM MN
Senior Lecturer
Ahilya Bai College of Nursing
Lok Nayak Hospital
New Delhi, India

Foreword
Saroj Kumar

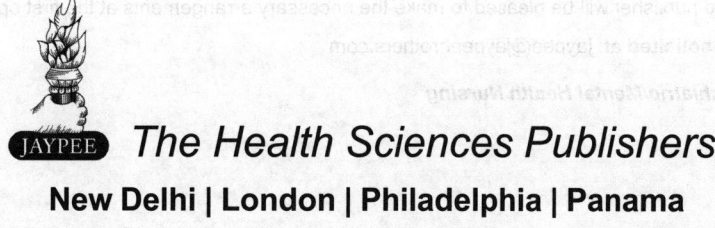

JAYPEE The Health Sciences Publishers
New Delhi | London | Philadelphia | Panama

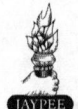 **Jaypee Brothers Medical Publishers (P) Ltd**

Headquarters
Jaypee Brothers Medical Publishers (P) Ltd
4838/24, Ansari Road, Daryaganj
New Delhi 110 002, India
Phone: +91-11-43574357
Fax: +91-11-43574314
Email: jaypee@jaypeebrothers.com

Overseas Offices

J.P. Medical Ltd
83 Victoria Street, London
SW1H 0HW (UK)
Phone: +44 20 3170 8910
Fax: +44 (0)20 3008 6180
Email: info@jpmedpub.com

Jaypee-Highlights Medical Publishers Inc
City of Knowledge, Bld. 237, Clayton
Panama City, Panama
Phone: +1 507-301-0496
Fax: +1 507-301-0499
Email: cservice@jphmedical.com

Jaypee Medical Inc.
The Bourse
111 South Independence Mall East
Suite 835, Philadelphia, PA 19106, USA
Phone: +1 267-519-9789
Email: jpmed.us@gmail.com

Jaypee Brothers Medical Publishers (P) Ltd
17/1-B Babar Road, Block-B, Shaymali
Mohammadpur, Dhaka-1207
Bangladesh
Mobile: +08801912003485
Email: jaypeedhaka@gmail.com

Jaypee Brothers Medical Publishers (P) Ltd
Bhotahity, Kathmandu
Nepal
Phone: +977-9741283608
Email: kathmandu@jaypeebrothers.com

Website: www.jaypeebrothers.com
Website: www.jaypeedigital.com

© 2015, Jaypee Brothers Medical Publishers

The views and opinions expressed in this book are solely those of the original contributor(s)/author(s) and do not necessarily represent those of editor(s) of the book.

All rights reserved. No part of this publication may be reproduced, stored or transmitted in any form or by any means, electronic, mechanical, photocopying, recording or otherwise, without the prior permission in writing of the publishers.

All brand names and product names used in this book are trade names, service marks, trademarks or registered trademarks of their respective owners. The publisher is not associated with any product or vendor mentioned in this book.

Medical knowledge and practice change constantly. This book is designed to provide accurate, authoritative information about the subject matter in question. However, readers are advised to check the most current information available on procedures included and check information from the manufacturer of each product to be administered, to verify the recommended dose, formula, method and duration of administration, adverse effects and contraindications. It is the responsibility of the practitioner to take all appropriate safety precautions. Neither the publisher nor the author(s)/editor(s) assume any liability for any injury and/or damage to persons or property arising from or related to use of material in this book.

This book is sold on the understanding that the publisher is not engaged in providing professional medical services. If such advice or services are required, the services of a competent medical professional should be sought.

Every effort has been made where necessary to contact holders of copyright to obtain permission to reproduce copyright material. If any have been inadvertently overlooked, the publisher will be pleased to make the necessary arrangements at the first opportunity.

Inquiries for bulk sales may be solicited at: jaypee@jaypeebrothers.com

Practical Record Book for Psychiatric/Mental Health Nursing

First Edition: 2008

Second Edition: 2015

Reprint **2024**

ISBN 978-93-5152-548-6

Printed at: Sterling Graphics Pvt. Ltd.

Foreword

Mental disorders have profound implications on the health and well-being not only of individuals but also of families and entire communities. The management of mentally ill is considered to be more challenging than other types of nursing care, because more than physical care the task involves interpersonal skills, sensitivity, knowledge of human behavior and interviewing skills. Therefore, it is essential to prepare nurses to care for mentally ill patients comprehensively.

This book is intended to provide guidelines and related notes to undergraduate student nurses undergoing psychiatric nursing clinical experience. It is broadly based on the guidance provided by Indian Nursing Council, which sets out the competencies the student nurses must reach on completion of their psychiatric nursing clinical experience. This book is particularly designed to help student nurses gain skill and the required competencies in dealing with mentally ill patients and providing them comprehensive nursing care.

Saroj Kumar
Vice-Principal
Ahilya Bai College of Nursing
Lok Nayak Hospital
New Delhi, India

Preface

Psychiatric Nursing is an essential component in the health care delivery system. During 1930–60, principles and practices of psychiatric nursing were derived from practical experiences of caring for psychiatric patients.

For years, students had been submitting assignments in loose sheets, and then later compiled it in a file, which sometimes gave a disorganized appearance. Thus, a need to prepare a record book for psychiatric/mental health nursing was felt by me. The writing of this practical record book is a sincere effort to organize the content and see that each student accomplishes what is required in a uniform manner.

The purpose of this book is to provide student nurses posted in psychiatric nursing care settings to fulfill the required clinical experience as per the Indian Nursing Council syllabus. This book comprises of two sections—Section-I and Section-II for III Year (VI Semester) and IV Year (Interns) undergraduate student nurses respectively. Section-I of this practical record book provides the related information/notes and the outlines for various assignments to be completed by the students during their psychiatric clinical experience postings. Section-II deals with assignments to be completed during their internship. The sequence and arrangements of the assignments according to sections or semesters can be changed by the user as per their convenience provided all the assignments are covered. Appendices are attached to help the students for ready reference to certain aspects, such as, classification, diagnoses, etc. Sample practical paper format is designed after years of practicing it successfully, and more or less similar format is used by examiners of different universities. Sample viva questions is just an effort to make viva more objective and that consistency is maintained while questioning students during viva.

My thanks are due to several people who motivated me in this venture, my teachers, colleagues and my ex-students. I dedicate this piece of my work to my beloved husband Late Mr Vipin Kishore Beck, who was my constant guide and driving force to bring out the second edition.

I thank Shri Jitendar P Vij (Group Chairman), Mr Ankit Vij (Group President) and Mr Tarun Duneja (Director-Publishing) of M/s Jaypee Brothers Medical Publishers (P) Ltd, New Delhi, India, for kindly agreeing to publish this book and accomplishing the task in a splendid manner. I also thank Mrs Samina Khan and Mr Subrata Adhikary, for their constant help and Mr Lalit Kumar, who did the secretarial job.

Last but not least, I thank my family members especially my sister Angela, my nephew Alvin and my sons Ronit and Eshaan, for their unending support and patience in helping me to complete this work.

I commend this publication to you and recommend that you use this practical record book, thereby ensuring that student nurses are supported and guided in a comprehensive manner while achieving competence to practice nursing safely and effectively.

Ellen Beck

Contents

SECTION-I: III-YEAR/VI SEMESTER

1. **Admission and Discharge** — 3
   Assignment 1: Admission 4
   Assignment 2: Discharge 7
2. **The Process of Assessing in Psychiatric/Mental Health Nursing Practice** — 9
   Assignment 3: History Taking 16
   Assignment 4: Mental Status Examination 31
   Assignment 5: Mini Mental State Examination 40
   Assignment 6: Investigations in Psychiatry 45
   Assignment 7: Neurological Examination 50
   Assignment 8: Psychological Tests 54
3. **The Nursing Process** — 57
   Assignment 9: Nursing Process/Care Plan 58
4. **Communication Techniques** — 73
   Assignment 10: Process Recording 76
5. **Case Presentation** — 109
   Assignment 11: Case Presentation 109
6. **Therapeutic Modalities** — 123
   Assignment 12: Electroconvulsive Therapy 124
   Assignment 13: Restraining 132
   Assignment 14: Psychopharmacology 139
   Assignment 15: Drug Presentation 193
   Assignment 16: Psychosocial Therapies 203
7. **Psychiatric OPD** — 208
   Assignment 17: History Taking 208
   Assignment 18: Mental Status Examination 213
   Assignment 19: Health Talk 221
   Assignment 20: Outpatient Department (OPD) 229
8. **Observation Reports** — 233
   Assignment 21: Child Guidance Clinic (CGC) 233
   Assignment 22: De Addiction Center 237
   Assignment 23: Occupational Therapy 241
9. **Evaluation of Clinical Performance** — 245

SECTION-II: IV-YEAR/VII SEMESTER

1. **Community Mental Health Nursing** — 249
   Assignment 1: Preventive Measures 249
   Assignment 2: Health Talk 253
   Assignment 3: Observation Report on Field Visit to a Mental Health Agency 261
2. **Project Work** — 267
   Assignment 4: Group Project 267
3. **Ward Administration** — 275
   Assignment 5: Ward Management of a Psychiatric Ward 275
4. **Evaluation of Clinical Performance** — 281

Bibliography — 283

Appendices — 285
  1. Nursing Diagnoses in Psychiatric Mental Health Nursing 285
  2. Classification of Mental Disorders 286
  3. CAGE 287
  4. Suicide Risk Assessment 288
  5. Sample Practical Examination Format 289
  6. Sample Viva Questions 290

Section 1

III-Year/VI Semester

1. Admission and Discharge
2. The Process of Assessing in Psychiatric/Mental Health Nursing Practice
3. The Nursing Process
4. Communication Techniques
5. Case Presentation
6. Therapeutic Modalities
7. Psychiatric OPD
8. Observation Reports
9. Evaluation of Clinical Performance

1 Admission and Discharge

ADMISSION

Overview

Hospitalization may be voluntary or involuntary. The client's safety, as well as the safety of others, is a critical factor in hospitalization. Conditions for hospitalization:
➢ Dangerous to oneself or others.
➢ Incapable of providing for one's basic physical needs.
➢ Unable to make reasonable decisions regarding hospitalization.
➢ In need of care or treatment in the hospital.

Types of Admission

The Mental Health Act (MHA), 1987 repeals Indian Lunacy Act, 1912 and Lunacy Act, 1977 (Jammu and Kashmir) and extends to whole of India. Under this Act, a mentally ill person means a person who is in need of treatment by reason of any mental disorder other than mental retardation.

Admission on Voluntary Basis

Any person aged eighteen and above can voluntarily get admission for inpatient treatment. In case of minor (less than 18 years of age) mentally ill, can be presented for admission by the guardian as a voluntary patient. However, the medical officer in-charge should be satisfied about the need for inpatient treatment.

Even though these hospital admissions are considered 'voluntary' they are regulated by states to ensure that:
1. Persons with mental disorders are sufficiently competent to make decisions of this kind,
2. In appropriate pressure or outfight coercion has not been exerted on a person already in custody to admit themselves, and
3. The person is truly willing to seek treatment therapy improving the prospects for success.

Admission Under Special Circumstances

Admission to psychiatric hospital under special circumstances can also be made on request of a relative or a friend of the patient if the patient is not in a position to express willingness for admission as a voluntary patient, provided the medical officer in-charge is satisfied that it is in interest of the patient to do so. This application should be accompanied by two medical certificates (one from a medical officer who is working in Government service) stating that the person has such mental illness that requires inpatient observation and treatment.

Admission Under a Reception Order

An application for reception order may be made by the medical officer in-charge of a mental hospital by the spouse or by any relative of the mentally ill patient for admission to the Magistrate. The application should be accompanied by two medical certificates from two independent medical practitioners certifying the need for admission for treatment and that it is in interest for personal safety of the patient or that of others. The consideration of the application should be made in the presence of applicant, the allegedly mentally ill person and the person appointed by the allegedly mentally ill to represent him. A reception order is valid up to 30 days or till discharged.

ASSIGNMENT 1: ADMISSION

1. Prepare an admission protocol for patients admitted in a psychiatric ward.

Admission and Discharge

DISCHARGE

Overview

Discharge planning begins when the client is admitted, whether it is the hospital, home care, or any other treatment program. The client, and when appropriate, the family must be involved in this process for it to be successful.

The patient who is *voluntarily admitted* to the hospital can leave at any time. The voluntarily admitted patient can be discharged by the staff when maximum benefit has been received from the treatment. Voluntary patients also may request discharge. Two key factors in deciding to release a voluntary psychiatric patient are:
- Assessment of the patient's competency.
- Assessment of the patient's potential danger to self or others.

An involuntarily admitted patient has lost the right to leave the hospital when he or she wishes. If a committed patient leaves before discharge, the staff has the legal obligation to notify the police and courts.

Discharge of Voluntary Patient

Patients admitted on voluntary basis, if they request for discharge, are obliged to be discharged by the medical officer in-charge within 24 hours of receiving the request, provided the medical officer is convinced that the discharge will not harm the interest of the voluntary patient. In such case, the medical officer would constitute a board of two medical officers and seek their opinion. If the board is of the opinion that such voluntary patient needs further treatment in the psychiatric hospital/psychiatric nursing home, the medical officer shall not discharge the voluntary patient but continue his treatment for a period not exceeding 90 days at a time.

Order of Discharge on the Undertaking of Relatives or Friends, etc. for Due Care of Mentally Ill Person

1. Where any relative or friend of a mentally ill person detained in a psychiatric hospital or psychiatric nursing home under section 22, 24 or 25 desires that such person shall be delivered over to his care and custody, he may make an application to the medical officer in-charge.
2. Where an application is received, the authority shall on such relative or friend furnishing a bond with or without sureties for such amount as such authority may specify in this behalf, undertaking to take proper care of such mentally-ill person, and ensuring that the mentally-ill person shall be prevented from causing injury to himself or to others, make an order of discharge and thereupon the mentally ill person shall be discharged.

Discharge of Person Subsequently Found on Inquisition to be of Sound Mind

If any person detained in a psychiatric hospital or nursing home in pursuance of a reception order made under this Act is subsequently found, on an inquisition, to be of sound mind is capable of taking care of himself and managing his affairs the medical officer in-charge shall forthwith on the production of a copy of such finding duly certified by the District Court, discharge such person from such hospital or nursing home.

Apart from admission and discharge detailed procedures have been laid down under various sections of the MHA for (to mention a few)

- Being taken into custody by the police, confinement and security of mentally ill persons or prisoners in a mental hospital.
- Ensuring proper care and custody to a mentally ill person by his legal relatives, through the police stations.
- For safety in hospital or during leave or absence or transfer to another hospital.
- Safe custody and protection of property of the patient.

Physical or mental cruelty to mentally ill patients is forbidden. Similarly conduct of research on a mentally ill patient is forbidden, unless voluntarily consent from patient or relative is obtained. The human rights of a mentally ill person are protected penalties and fines for contravening the provisions of the Act have been discussed in various sections of the MHA.

ASSIGNMENT 2: DISCHARGE

1. Discuss discharge summary of your patient and nurses responsibility.

2 | The Process of Assessing in Psychiatric/Mental Health Nursing Practice

OVERVIEW

The psychiatric nursing assessment provides an opportunity for the nurse to gather data to be used in treatment of the client. Specific information about the client's thoughts, feelings and behavior is obtained. In addition, the environmental stimuli that affect these thoughts, feelings and behavior are investigated.

The most widely used assessment tool is the psychiatric interview. The assessment may be completed in a single, initial interview or in several interviews. Assessment is used to elicit sufficient information to identify problems and to formulate beginning plans for intervention.

THE PSYCHIATRIC INTERVIEW

Definition

The interview is a purposeful, goal directed interaction in which the nurse builds an alliance with the client while collecting data for assessment.

Types

Two types of interviews are used in a psychiatric setting:
   a. **Fact finding:** It is conducted to help the nurse gain specific knowledge about an event. In this type of interview, the nurse has a goal to elicit specific data from the patient. There usually is a preset group of questions that are asked to the patient, e.g. mental status examination.
   b. **One to one interaction:** The second type of interview is referred to as the nurse-patient relationship or one to one interaction. This interview is useful in allowing the patient time to explore problems that have been unresolved upto that point. In this type of interview, the nurse and patient together identify and work on problems that, when resolved will help the patient function in a more adaptive and effective manner, e.g. process recording.

Purposes

1. The overall purpose of the interview is to provide a database of information from which the nurse and patient together can identify problems, set goals and evaluate methods of achieving the goals that have been set.

2. The interview becomes a vehicle for helping the patient move towards emotional health.
3. The interview is also a valuable tool in helping students become comfortable in talking with patients.
4. The interview is useful in providing an opportunity for the patient to establish a meaningful relationship with the student.

ESSENTIALS OF AN INTERVIEW

Time

Generally, the time should not exceed one hour. For patients who are actually disturbed, severely regressed or suffering from organic impairment, the interview should be informal and brief (5–10 minutes) until the patient is well enough to tolerate regular meetings of increasing periods of time.

Place

For the interview to be successful, the patient should be seen in a quiet place. It is distracting to try to talk in a busy ward where many patients are walking about and are likely to interrupt the interaction. Concern for privacy is vitally important.

Comfort

Your own comfort during an interview is essential in order to hear what the patient is saying and to be receptive to what the patient is having difficulty expressing. For example, when you are hungry, tired or preoccupied, you are not going to be a good listener. At the same time, be sure that the time and place of meeting are acceptable to the client. He will be unable to respond effectively if he is hungry, sleepy or unsure of the purpose of the interview.

SKILLS OF THE NURSE INTERVIEWER

A client usually prefers an active, friendly interviewer who verbalized minimally and uses effective communication techniques. The key elements in facilitative communication include the following:

- **Active listening:** It focuses on the patient's verbal and non-verbal communication and by being alert and open without projecting one's own values and ideas on the client.
- **Concreteness:** It refers to specificity of communication and persistence in requesting the client to describe feelings and events in specific terms rather than vague or abstract terms.
- **Immediacy:** It refers to the interviewer's ability to recognize feelings and thoughts which are of immediate importance to the client and to deal with those issues first.
- **Experiential confrontation:** It involves the interviewer's consistently pointing out discrepencies and generalizations during the interview.
- **Didactic confrontation:** It occurs when the interviewer objectively offers the client relevant informatin to correct misinformation.

RECORDING INTERVIEW

Recording of data gathered during the interview can be completed in a variety of ways, depending on the needs and wishes of the client and nurse.

One method is for the interviewer to keep a **verbatim** written recording. This method allows accuracy, but disrupts the flow of the interview process.

Another method of recording is to use a third person nonparticipant to record the verbatim interview conversation and to note, as much as possible, the nonverbal communication. The presence of the third person, however, may significantly alter the dynamics of the interview, particularly trust, and may be perceived as a violation of psychological privacy.

Probably the most widely used approach is the recording of brief notes throughout the interview or the making of "**mental notes**," followed by writing of a summary of verbal and nonverbal data later. Although, this method offers greater comfort for the client, it may not provide optimal accuracy.

Audio and video tape recordings are the most reliable methods of recording during the interview. Videotaping allows a review of the session and gives the most complete information about the client's communication within the environmental context. Before planning to tape record an interview the nurse must ascertain that institutional policies permit taping and that the client has given his approval by signing a permission form. Problems related to taping an interview include client discomfort, irritation and suspicion.

Recording of assessment information including a thorough client history, description of the problem, and the client's abilities and potential sources of motivation, allows for an accurate analysis of the data. Gathering client assessment data enables the nurse to formulate accurate diagnoses, which form the bases for nursing care plans.

PSYCHOSOCIAL HISTORY

The collecting of the patient's history is of fundamental importance, both for investigation and for treatment.

The history when completed should give a picture of the patient's development and adjustment during his life. It should contain relevant information on possible genetic and family influences on his personality and his illness. It should portray his development from childhood to adult life. It should provide evidence of adjustment to school, work, marriage, society together with a record of his physical and mental health and previous personality.

The psychosocial history is better understood if it is organized into identifying data, chief complaint, present problem and past personal history.

IDENTIFYING DATA

Identification — includes the basic demographics of the patient:

Name:	Ward:
Age:	Bed no.:
Sex:	CR no.:
Race:	Date of admission:

Marital status:
Number and ages of children/siblings:
Spouse/parents ages (still living):
Living arrangements:
Occupation:

Education:
Religion:					Nationality					Native place:
Mother tongue:
Address:
Brought by/informant:
Diagnosis/Provisional Diagnosis

CHIEF COMPLAINT

The chief complaint is a verbatim recording of the patient's reason for seeking treatment or evaluation or the presenting problem for which the client is seeking professional help. The chief complaints should be stated in the client's own words.

HISTORY OF THE PRESENT ILLNESS

It is a chronological description of how symptoms in the current episode have unfolded over time.
History of the present problem can also be collected by the informant.
- When did the problem begin?
- How does the client describe his symptoms?
- What has happened recently to upset the client? The amount of stress the client has been recently experiencing can be estimated by using the Holmes and Rahe social readjustment rating scale. An accumulation of 200 or more life change units in 1 year can trigger a physical or psychiatric problem.
- Has there been a change in somatic functioning—Sleep disturbance, appetite or weight change or change in sexual interest or performance?
- Has there been a change in the client's mental status—feelings of anxiety or depression?

PERSONAL HISTORY

It describes events of major significance throughout a person's life. Major items commonly include early childhood friendships, education, any changes in school performance, romantic involvements, work history, jail experiences and leisure activities. Personal history can be collected under the following headings:

A. Infancy

- Was the pregnancy full term?
- Did the client's mother experience prenatal difficulties or problems during labor and delivery?
- Was the client breastfed or bottle fed?
- What was the age of passing important developmental milestones?
- Are there any memories of toilet training, motor development or early or delayed use of language?
- Did the client's mother use drugs or alcohol during pregnancy?
- Whether the patient was brought up by mother or someone else and any history suggestive of maternal deprivation.

B. Childhood

- Which childhood diseases or hospitalizations occurred?
- How would he describe his relationships with each of his parents?
- How did he adjust to school and peers?
- Was there any child abuse or sexual abuse?
- Did his parents drink? How much?
- What games did he play with whom and where?
- The presence of neurotic traits to be noted like stammering, stuttering, tics, thumb sucking, nail biting, head banging, rocking, night terrors, phobias, temper tantrums, etc.

C. Adolescence

- How did the client react to the onset of puberty?
- How did his parents react?
- Did he feel adequately prepared for the maturational changes?
- How did he relate to his family?
- Was he over complaint or aggressively rebellious?
- How did he relate to his peers?
- Did he feel part of the "in group" or isolated and different?
- How did he react to any sexual experimentation?
- Was there acting out behavior involving drugs, sex, or truancy or difficulties with breaking the law?

D. Adulthood

- What level of education did the client achieve?
- Does he feel that he has accomplished his educational objectives?

Work History

- What is his work history? (It includes summary of jobs held, length of time in each and the reasons for leaving.)
- Does he feel satisfied with his work?
- Was there interruption of education or work owing to physical or psychological difficulties?

Marital History

Information regarding duration of marriage, arranged marriage or by self choice, with or without parents consent, number of marriages, divorces or separation, role in marriage can be asked.

Sexual History

- What is his sexual orientation or preference?
- Does he feel comfortable with his sexual/marital relationship?

- Is there any sexual dysfunction?
- If client is a female, has there been any difficulty conceiving, pregnancies or abortion?

Deteriorating school performance, an irregular work history with failure to progress to higher levels of responsibility, an inability to sustain friendships or romantic involvement for any period of time all may have diagnostic and prognostic significance. The personal history also helps, identify key events that may have helped precipitate current symptoms like divorce, death, loss of work, financial set backs. However, with the exception of PTSD identification of a precipitating event is not required to make a diagnosis.

E. Medical History

- Has the client experienced any significant illness, injury or surgery?
- Did he require hospitalization?
- How did he react to the illness or hospitalization?
- Is he taking any prescribed or illicit drug?
- Does he have any allergies?
- Has he experienced any significant side effect of psychotropic medications?

The occurrence of major illness or surgery is likely to be of considerable significance in a person's life and may be a precipitant of psychiatric disturbance. For example, a middle aged man following a heart attack may develop anxiety, depression and a fear for sex.

F. Family History

A family history shows who is in the family, who is available for support, who may be exacerbating symptoms, whether a general vulnerability of psychiatric disorders exists and what stresses have been caused by a family member's illness.

- Who constitutes the client's nuclear family, extended family and family of origin?
- Was he an only child, the youngest or oldest child?
- Were there breakdowns in the family unit due to separation, divorce, or death?
- Is there a history of physical or psychiatric illness in family members?
- Is there a history of suicide attempts or completed suicide, alcoholism, or child abuse?
- Is there a history of extramarital relationship?

Also see appendix 4-suicide risk assessment.

Genogram

A genogram is a pictorial representation of at least three generations of a family. In a genogram, the names of the family members are placed on horizontal lines to indicate separate generations. Vertical lines denote children. The children are ranked from oldest to youngest, going from left to right. A family is often interested in doing a genogram because it gives them a diagram of family relationships, including significant information (Fig. 2.1).

G. Past Psychiatric History

It describes all previous episodes and symptoms whether treated or not. Many psychiatric disorders are familial and many of those appear to have a genetic component to the cause.

The Process of Assessing in Psychiatric/Mental Health Nursing Practice

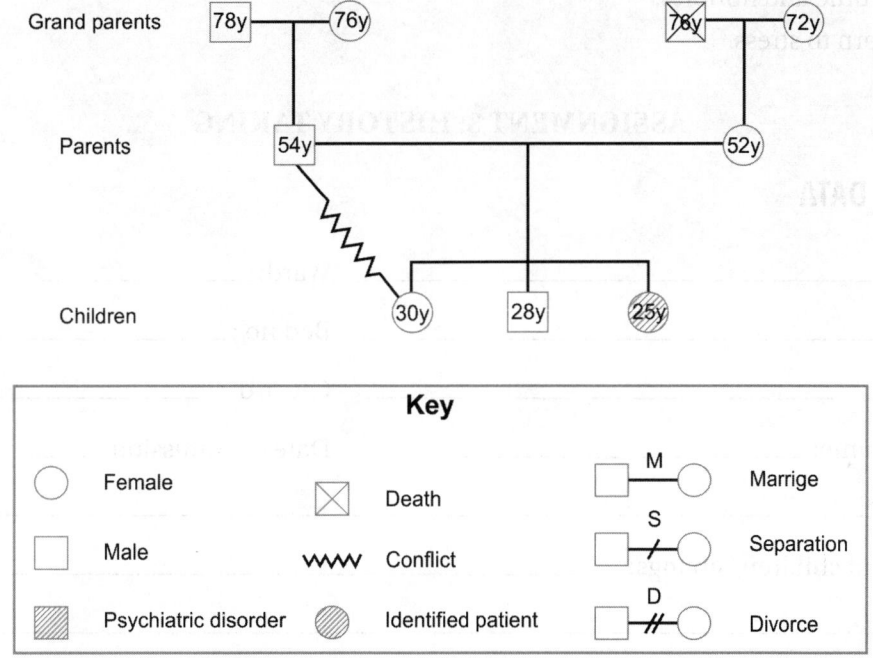

Fig. 2.1: Sample three generation genogram

- Has the client received any psychiatric treatment in the past?
- Has he been hospitalized for this treatment?
- What medications were prescribed?
- Did he receive electroconvulsive therapy?
- What were the results of any treatment modality? In this, the therapeutic benefits and adverse effects can be noted.

Substance Use

- Determine the last use of alcohol and illicit or abused drugs and the amount.
- Ask when did he/she started using it more than intended.
- Any past history of substance use.
  Also See Appendix-3 CAGE in case to assess for alcoholism.

H. Premorbid Personality

It refers to the personality of the individual prior to illness. Information can be collected to access this in the following areas:
- Social relations with friends, family members, colleagues, neighbors.
- Attitude towards self-self concept.
- Predominant mood.
- Religious and moral beliefs.
- Fantasies—day dreams, amount of time spent day dreaming.

- Use of leisure time and hobbies.
- Reaction pattern to stress.

ASSIGNMENT 3: HISTORY TAKING

IDENTIFICATION DATA

Name: _____   Ward: _____

Age: _____   Bed no.: _____

Sex: _____   CR no.: _____

Father/husband name: _____   Date of admission: _____

Marital status: _____

Number and ages of children/siblings: _____

Spouse/parents age: _____

Living arrangements: _____

Occupation: _____

Education: _____

Religion: _____   Nationality: _____

Mother tongue: _____

Address: _____

Brought by/informant: _____

Diagnosis/provisional diagnosis: _____

CHIEF COMPLAINTS: _____

_____

_____

_____

_____

_____

_____

HISTORY OF PRESENT ILLNESS:

PERSONAL HISTORY:

Infancy:

Childhood:

Adolescence: ___

Adulthood: ___

MEDICAL HISTORY:

FAMILY HISTORY:

GENOGRAM:

PAST PSYCHIATRIC HISTORY:

PREMORBID PERSONALITY:

ANY OTHER SPECIAL POINT:

The Process of Assessing in Psychiatric/Mental Health Nursing Practice

MENTAL STATUS EXAMINATION

Overview

The mental status examination is analogous to the physical examination in physical medicine. It provides a format for the systematic observation and recording of information about a person's thinking, emotions and behavior.

The elements of the examination depends on the patient's clinical presentation, as well as his educational and cultural background. It also serves as a basis for future comparison to facilitate tracking in the patients program over time. The examination itself is usually divided into several parts. Some parts of the mental status examination are assessed by observing the client's facial expression and sense of grooming. Other aspects require asking questions to assess cognitive functioning.

Definition

- Mental status examination is a way of organizing observational data about all aspects of a patient's mental functioning.
- Mental status examination is an organized systematic approach to assessment of an individuals current psychiatric condition.

Purposes

The performance and recording of a mental status examination have several major functions:
1. It is an agreed upon method of organizing clinical observations.
2. It provides a clinical baseline for a patient's psychological state.
3. It provides specific information that assists in establishing certain diagnoses.

GENERAL APPEARANCE

A brief description is given of the patient's appearance, behavior and manner of relating to the examiner. With particular attention paid to abnormalities, special attention needs to be paid to grooming, dress, facial expressions, posture and gait.

A. Grooming

- Is the patient taking care of his/her appearance?
- What is the appearance of the teeth, hair, nails, body?
- If a woman patient uses cosmetic make up, is it done appropriately for the situation?

B. Dress

- Is the dress appropriate for the season and situation?
  Manic patients may dress in colorful or unusual attire.

C. Facial Expression

- What is the patient's facial expression?
- Impassive, expressionless, excited, sad, angry, startled, suspicious, grimacing?

The Process of Assessing in Psychiatric/Mental Health Nursing Practice

➤ Does the patient avoid eye contact stare at the examiner, look around the room, stare down or into space? Dilated pupils are sometimes associated with drug intoxication. Constricted pupils indicate narcotic addiction.

D. Posture and Gait

➤ How does the patient sit in the chair?
➤ Erect, slumped down on the edge of the chair, leaning forward, backward on his/her elbows?
➤ When the patient walks, does he/she move quickly, slowly, with hesitation, a limp, head erect or hung down? Stooped posture is often seen in patients with depression.

SPEECH

The nurse can assess several aspects of the client's form of speech.

A. Volume

➤ How loudly or softly does the client speak?
➤ Does the examiner have to adjust his/her position to hear?

B. Rate

➤ What is the speed of the patient's speech?
➤ Rapid with very few pauses?
➤ Or are there long pauses between words?

C. Tone

➤ Is there a wide range in the pitch of the voice sounds?
➤ Is the sound of his voice boring, tedious or monotonous?

D. Productivity

➤ Are the questions answered in one word responses a. yes or no?
➤ Are details offered?
➤ Are questions expanded?
➤ Do simple questions yield complex or overly detailed responses?

E. Goal Direction

➤ Do the answers follow a logical sequence?
➤ Do the answers make sense?
➤ Does the focus remain clear?

F. Pitch

➤ Is the voice shrieky or thick?

G. Reaction Time

➤ How long the patient takes to answer any question?

Abnormalities of Speech

1. Qualitative.
2. Quantitative.
3. Both.

Qualitative Abnormalities

- **Circumstantiality:** The person digresses into unnecessary details and unusual thoughts before saying the central idea. Person includes needless peripheral details (often seen in schizophrenia).
- **Perseveration:** Repetition of same response to different questions (often indicates organic involvement).
- **Irrelevance:** A rational statement but not germane (relevant or pertinent).
- **Incoherence:** Difficult to follow or understand the patient due to impairment in the manner of speech.
- **Word salad:** An incoherent mixture of words (often seen in schizophrenia).
- **Neologism:** Invention of new words or condensation of words (seen in psychotic disorders) or use of conventional words in idiosyncratic ways.
- **Echolalia:** A pathological repetition of words used by one person.
- *Verbigeration*: Senseless repetition of words or phrases over and over again.

Quantitative Abnormalities

- Pressurized talk (as seen in mania).
- Scanty talk or using only monosyllabic talk (as seen in mutism or depression)
    - Mutism is refusal to speak (as seen in psychotic patients).

Any other abnormality like stammering, stuttering, dysarthria or aphasia should also be noted.

MOTOR BEHAVIOR

The nurse should assess for posture, gait, tics, tremors, posturing grimaces and other abnormal bodily movements. The speed of these movements is important to note.

- Is there a general slowness of movement?
- Does these appear to be much effort expended just to talk, walk or gesture?
- Or do the movements appear to be intense and rapid?
- The behaviors that include nail biting, wringing of the hands, tapping of the foot, and chewing movements may be clues to the individual's anxiety and an increase or decrease of these behaviors can be noted as the interview progresses and deals with emotionally charged material.

Abnormal Motor Behavior

- **Echopraxia:** The pathological repetition by imitation of the movements of another person.
- *Waxy flexibility* or cerea flexibility in which persons can hold his body in one position for a long period of time (as see in catatonic schizophrenia).
- **Catalepsy:** A generalized condition of diminished responsiveness often is characterized by trance like states and immobility (as seen in depression).

- **Cataplexy:** A temporary loss of muscle tone and may be precipitated by surprise, laughter or anger (as seen in schizophrenia).
- **Compulsion:** An insistent, repetitive intrusive and unwanted urge to act in a way contrary to one's usual wishes or standards.
- **Mania:** The suffix mania is used with Greek terms to indicate a preoccupation with certain kinds of activities or a compulsive need to behave abnormally, e.g.
    - Egomania—Pathological preoccupation with self.
    - Kleptomania—The compulsion to steal.
    - Megalomania—Pathological preoccupation with delusions of power/wealth.
    - Necromania—Pathological preoccupation with dead bodies.
    - Pyromania—Morbid compulsion to set fires.

ATTITUDE

The attitude of the client may be assessed by observing if he is cooperative, evasive, arrogant, ingratiating, spontaneous, assertive or withdrawn during the interview.
- What is the client's attitude about coming to the clinic or hospital?
- Toward the interview?
- Towards his illness or problem?
- These observations provide clues regarding patterns of relating to people as well as clues to the client's defense mechanisms. For example, attitudes denoting suspiciousness, evasiveness and arrogance may indicate paranoid patterns; an uncooperative or impatient attitude may indicate manic patterns; a remote, reserved or uninvolved attitude may indicate a schizophrenic pattern; an apprehensive worrisome attitude may reflect neurotic pattern; an overly confident, ingratiating attitude may indicate a personality disorder; an apathetic detached attitude may indicate depression; and an easily distracted, seemingly indifferent attitude may indicate a person suffering from an acute brain disorder.

EMOTIONAL EXPRESSION

Emotional expression is described in terms of mood and affect.

Mood

A pervasive and sustained emotion that colors the person's perception of the world. Mood is the patient's self-report of the prevailing emotional state. Mood can be assessed by asking simple questions like "how are you feeling today". The individuals' subjective description of his feeling is his mood. Ask the client to describe his mood. Have there been any mood changes noted. If so were these changes in mood rapid, cyclic or situational? Assess the client's dominant mood during the interview, i.e. depressed, anxious, angry. There are many possible moods: depression, elation, euphoria, anger, suspicion, fear, anxiety, panic hostility, calm, happiness, sadness, grief and a combination of these.

If the potential for suicide is suspected, the nurse should ask about the patients thought about self-harm. Suicidal and homicidal thoughts must be addressed directly. To judge the patient's suicidal or homicidal risk, the nurse should assess the patient's plans, ability to carry out plans, patient's attitude about death and any support system available.

Affect

The outward expression of the patients inner experiences. It refers to what the individual is feeling at the moment—the emotional state and outward appearance. Several areas can be noted when assessing affect. Affect can be described in terms of the following:

Range
- **Limited/narrow:** Only a few emotions are expressed.
- **Wide/labile:** Frequent shifts between very different emotions, e.g. laughing, crying (often seen in mania).
- **Blunting:** Leads to flattening (no response at all).

Intensity: The quality of emotion expressed.
- Flat with little energy or exaggerated with great energy.

Types: Different kind/categories of emotions—sad, fearful, happy, angry, elated, etc.

Appropriateness: Does the affect expressed fit the outcome expressed?
- **Appropriate affect:** A young woman is crying and fearful as she describes an attempted rape.
- **Inappropriate affect:** A 40-years-old man smiles when describing how angry he is at his father (also called bizarre affect).
- **Incongruence:** When there is no association between thought and emotion. For example, a patient reports being persecuted by the police and then laughs.
- **Bland or flat affect:** Emotional tone is very weak, appears to be void of emotional tone/response.
- **Apathy:** Apathy is a term that may be used to describe an individual's display of lack of emotion, interest or concern in the environment. The bland or flat affect is a manifestation of emotional apathy.

PERCEPTION

Perception is the capacity to be aware of objects and to discriminate between them. Three major perception disorders are:
1. Illusion.
2. Hallucination.
3. Depersonalization and Derealization.

Illusion

The misperception of some real external sensory experience/stimulus, such as noise or shadows. For example, patient looks outside the window and sees a shadow of a tree as a real person and hears the wind calling his name. Illusions are widely believed to be more common in delirium than in other psychiatric disorders.

Hallucination

It is a false sensory perception in the absence of external stimuli. Hallucinations may have different origins, such as psychosis, a brain tumor, drug reaction, drug-alcohol overdose, sleep deprivation and hepatic failure.

There may be vague sounds, flashes of light or recognizable voices, faces, insects or odors. It may involve any of the sense organ. They can occur in any sensory modality.
- **Visual** — Hallucination of sight
- **Auditory** — Hallucination of sound
- **Olfactory** — Hallucination of smell
- **Tactile** — Hallucination of touch
- **Gustatory** — Hallucination of taste
- **Visceral** — Hallucination of sensation.

Command Hallucinations are those that tell the patient to do something such as kill one-self, harm another, etc.

Auditory hallucinations are the most common. In evaluating them one should ask the patient to identify the voice and sex of the person, also is the voice friendly or threatening? What is the voice saying to the patient?

The modality of hallucination has no diagnostic significance, with the exception of **formication** a tactile hallucination of insects crawling over or under the skin, which is strongly associated with withdrawal from alcohol and sedatives.

Depersonalization

A feeling that one is outside of one's body. This often is accompanied by a **derealization** in which the person feels a kind of strangeness about his immediate surroundings almost like being in a dream. (the sense that oneself or the world as not real).

THINKING

Attention is paid to the content of the client's speech, observations may be made regarding disturbances in the thought process, structure and rate of association and in the flow of ideas.

Thinking is subdivided into two sub-categories: Form and content.

Thought Form

Thought form refers to the way in which ideas are linked not the ideas themselves.

Does the client's thinking and communication proceed in a relatively clear, understandable manner? For example, abnormalities include:
- **Circumstantiality:** Over inclusion of trivial or tireless details that impede the sense of getting to the point.
- **Incoherence**
- **Neologisms**
- **Word salad**
- **Echolalia**
- **Perseveration**
- **Thought blocking:** A sudden disruption of thought or break, in the flow of ideas sudden stopping in the middle of a sentence with no understanding of why.
- **Loose association:** Lack of logical order in content. It is synonymous with derailment.
- **Condensation:** One symbol stands for a number of other and results in the fusion of various ideas into one.

- **Flight of ideas:** Describes a succession of thought without logical connections. Thought seem to move abruptly from idea to idea.
- **Retardation:** The slowly down of thought processes.
- **Tangentiality:** Differs from circumstantiality in that the person never really gets to the point of the communication. Unrelated topics are introduced and the original discussion is lost.
- **Clang association:** Thought are associated by the sound of words rather than their meaning.

Thought Content

Thought content describes a patient's ideas. It should be assessed by listening carefully to the patient's pre-occupations, ambitions and dreams. By assessing the major themes and issues discussed by the patient the nurse can identify the dominant themes that the patient is expressing. Does the patient relate most of what he considers his difficulty to a sense of failure, fear of harm, loss of an important person, phobias, fear of loosing impulse control or certain ritualistic compulsive behavior? An important area to be assessed is the suicidal and homicidal ideation.

Abnormalities of content include delusions, preoccupations, phobias and obsessions.

Delusion

It is a false, fixed, firm idea, not shared by others and which is inconsistent with the client's educational and cultural background or which cannot be corrected. Types of delusions:
- **Persecutory delusion:** Person believes that there is an organized conspiracy to hurt or harm him in some way.
- **Paranoid delusions:** It includes ideas of persecution, suspiciousness, megalomanic, grandiose notions, e.g. CBI is out to kill me.
- **Somatic/hypochondria delusion:** Person is certain that his body is deteriorating from within or that someone is in his brain. Person has ideas of bodily changes, e.g. feeling that their internal organs have changed into stones, bowels have disappeared, rats are eating up their brains.
- **Delusion of grandeur:** Person believes that he is a famous or an important person, i.e. God, PM, CM, etc.
- **Delusion of guilt:** Person believes that his bad thoughts have power to affect or influence others.
- **Influence/ideas of control:** Person believes that his thoughts are being controlled by objects/person outside of himself, e.g. superman power—my thoughts are controlling PM.
- **Thought broadcasting:** Patient believes that one's thoughts are being aired to the outside world.
- **Ideas of reference:** The patient who believes that everyday neutral occurrences carry specific unique and personal significance is said to have ideas of reference, e.g. a person may believe that a television announcer is attempting to convey a hidden message or that a stranger passing by on the street is signaling something. For example, I could see them talking about me.
- **Nihilistic Delusion:** Delusion of negation, believes he has done some harm to someone near.
- **Delusion of self-accusation.**

Preoccupation

Preoccupations are thoughts that predominate a person's thinking but are usually not experienced as unwanted or symptomatic. For example, include preoccupation with health, money or social status or with injustices.

The Process of Assessing in Psychiatric/Mental Health Nursing Practice

Phobias

They are persistent, unrealistic obsessive fear or dread of an object or situation held by a person.

Major phobias are:
- Acrophobia — fear of heights
- Agoraphobia — fear of open places
- Claustrophobia — fear of closed spaces
- Pyrophobia — fear of fire
- Panophobia — fear of everything
- Algophobia — fear of pain
- Zoophobia — fear of animal
- Xenophobia — fear of strangers.

Obsession

Obsessions are unwanted, intrusive thoughts experienced by patients as symptomatic and beyond their control. Repeated ideas coming to a person's mind in spite of knowing, it is illogical. The content of an obsession may be virtually anything but it is often a disturbing thought of doing something embarrassing, hurtful or dangerous.

SENSORIUM AND COGNITION

Assessment of various cognitive functions that collectively describes the overall intactness of the CNS.

1. **Alertness**
   - Alertness describes the degree of wakefulness and may range from fully awake and alert to comatose and non-responsiveness.
   - How alert the patient is? It may be transient—as in toxic states for a short time or permanent—as in dementia for a long time.
2. **Orientation:** Assessment of client regarding—orientation to time, place and person.
   - Time—does the patient know the time or day of the week, month, year?
   - Place—does the patient know where he is, where he lives, how he got to where he presently is?
   - Person—does the patient know who he is, who is with him, name.
3. **Concentration:** Concentration describes the ability to sustain attention over time.
   i. Focus of responses—does patient have difficulty in focusing his answers? Is the patient easily distracted?
   ii. Simple calculation—can patient perform simple math additions, subtractions, etc.?

   Test for Level of Concentration
   - Add any two small whole numbers.
   - Name the days of the week backwards.
   - Perform a "serial threes" or serial sevens test—that is subtract 3 from 100 or 7 from 100 until he reaches 0 for a substantial period of time.
   - Name the months of the year backwards.
   - Reciting the alphabets backwards.
4. **Memory** must be evaluated across the spectrum of immediate to remote.
   a. **Immediate recall:** Recall of information or data to which a person was just exposed to. Say a series of numbers and have the patient repeat the series within a 10 second internal.

b. **Recent:** Recall of events, information and people from the past week or so. Recent memory is for events several minutes to hours old and may be evaluated by giving patients the names of 3-4 unrelated object and asking them to repeat them after 5-10 minutes. Can he remember the events of last week, what he had for breakfast?

   Disorder of recent memory: Anterograde amnesia is the absence of memory for recent events.

c. **Remote:** Recall of events, information and people from the distant past. Remote memory describes events 2 or more years old. It is usually revealed in the course of obtaining patients' histories. Can he remember his birthday, marriage, etc. things of past disorder. Retrograde amnesia is the absence of memory for past events.

5. **Ability to Abstract:** Abstract reasoning describes the ability to mentally shift back and forth between general concepts and specific examples. One of the frequent ways to test abstract reasoning is asking proverb interpretation.

   ➤ Ask the patient to state the meaning of proverbs, e.g. do not cry over spilt milk, A stitch in time saves nine.
   ➤ One alternative to proverb interpretation in assessing abstract reasoning is to ask for similarity between two or more items.
   ➤ Ask the patient to describe the similarity between the objects in each of the pairs below, e.g.
      – An apple and an orange
      – A chair and a table.

6. **Insight:** It is the capacity of the patient to recognize and understand their own symptoms and illness.
   – Does the patient recognizes that he is having emotional or mental problems.
   – What is his/her level of motivation to work on his difficulties?
   – Is he aware of how his difficulties affect his life in general?

   Insight is rated on a 6 point scale from 1 to 6.
   a. Complete denial of illness.
   b. Slight awareness being sick.
   c. Awareness of being sick attributed it to external of physical labor.
   d. Awareness of being sick but due to something unknown in himself.
   e. Intellectual insight.
   f. True emotional insight.

7. **Judgment:** The nurse assesses the client's judgment by observing his ability to make and carry out plans, to take the initiative, to discriminate accurately and to behave according to accepted practice. To test for such a process, the nurse can ask such questions as:

   "What would you do if you found a stamped envelope in the street? Explain why criminals are put in prison. Describe what you would do if stopped for speeding? Assessment can be made as to the judgment is logical or illogical.

8. **Fund of knowledge:** Fund of knowledge must be tailored to the unique circumstances and educational level of the individual. Patients are often asked to name the president, questions about current events, key geographical facts (oceans, rivers) and sports may further help in assessment. It depends on the level of formal education, it gives an estimate of the patient's intellectual capabilities. Questions should have relevance to the patient's educational and cultural background.

Sometimes intelligence is advocated in the MSE. This cannot be done with any validity or reliability without the use of standardized instruments, and even then it may be difficult to distinguish between intelligence and education.

ASSIGNMENT 4: MENTAL STATUS EXAMINATION

1. Identification data

Name: _____ Ward: _____

Age: _____ Bed no.: _____

Sex: _____ CR no.: _____

Father/husband name: _____ Date of admission: _____

Marital status: _____

Number and ages of children/siblings: _____

Spouse/parents age: _____

Living arrangements: _____

Occupation: _____

Education: _____

Religion: _____ Nationality: _____

Mother tongue: _____

Address: _____

Brought by/informant: _____

Diagnosis/provisional diagnosis: _____

2. General description

General appearance _____
_____
_____
_____
_____
_____
_____

Speech

Motor behavior

Attitude

3. Emotional expression

Mood _____

Affect _____

4. Experiences

Perception _____

_____

_____

_____

_____

_____

_____

_____

_____

_____

_____

5. Thinking

Thought form _____

_____

_____

_____

Thought content _____

_____

_____

_____

_____

6. Sensorium and cognition

Alertness _____

_____

_____

_____

Orientation

Concentration

Memory

Ability to abstract

Insight

Judgment

Fund of knowledge

7. Any other special point

MINI MENTAL STATE EXAMINATION

At times, it is not practical to complete a full mental status examination. On these occasions nurses find it easy to use mini-mental status examination (Folstein, Folstein and McHugh 1975). It is the simplified score form of the cogniture mental status examination. It consists of few questions and requires only five to 10 minutes to administer.

Components	Time Allowed (Seconds)	Score
I. **Orientation** (maximum score 10)		
1. What year is this?	10	1
2. What season is this?	10	1
3. What months is this?	10	1
4. What is today's date?	10	1
5. What day of the weak is this?	10	1
6. What country are we in?	10	1
7. Which state are we in?	10	1
8. Which city/town are we in?	10	1
9. In home—What is the street address of this house?	10	1
10. In hospital—What is the name of this building	10	1
II. **Registration** (Maximum score 3)		
SAY—I am going to name three objects, when I am finished, I want you to repeat them. Remember what they are because I am going to ask you to name them again in a few minutes. Say the following words slowly at 01 second interval ball/car/man. Give one point for each correct answer.	20	3
III. **Attention and calculation** (Maximum score 5)	—	
Ask the client to begin at 100 and count backwards by 7. Stop after 5 subtractions (93, 86, 79, 72, 65). Give one point for each correct number or If the client cannot perform this task ask him/her to spell the word now spell it backwards. Give one point for each correctly placed letter.	3	5
IV. **Recall** (Maximum score 3)	10	3
Say what are the three objects I had asked you to remember		
V. **Language** (Maximum score 9)		
Naming	10	1
– Show wrist watch. Ask what is this?		
– Show pencil. Ask what is this?	10	1
Repetition	10	1
– Say I would like you to repeat this phrase after me. No ifs, ands or buts.		
Three stage command	30	3
– Give the subject a piece of blank paper and say. "Take the paper in your right hand fold it in half and put it on the floor. Give one point for each action performed correctly.		

Contd...

Contd...

Components	Time Allowed (Seconds)	Score
Reading On a blank piece of paper print the sentence. "Close your eyes." SAY—read the words on the page and then do what it says. Score correctly only if he/she actually closes his/her eyes.	10	1
Writing Hand the person a pencil and paper. SAY—write any complete sentence on the piece of paper (The sentence must make sense, ignore spelling errors).	30	1
Copying Place design, eraser and pencil in front of the person. SAY—copy this design please. Figure Allow multiple tries. Want until the person has finished and hands it back. All 10 angles need to be present and the two shapes must interest to score 1 point.	60	1
Total		30

Maximum score 30, score < 20 suggests significant cognitive impairment.
Source: Folstein, Folstein and McHugh

ASSIGNMENT 5: MINI MENTAL STATE EXAMINATION

1. Identification data

Name: _____ Ward: _____

Age: _____ Bed no.: _____

Sex: _____ CR no.: _____

Father/husband name: _____ Date of admission: _____

Marital status: _____

Number and ages of children/siblings: _____

Spouse/parents age: _____

Living arrangements: _____

Occupation: _____

Education: _____

Religion: _____ Nationality: _____

Mother tongue: _____

Address: _____

Brought by/informant: _____

Diagnosis/provisional diagnosis: _____

Components	Time Allowed (Seconds)	Score
I. **Orientation** (maximum score 10)		
1. What year is this?	10	
2. What season is this?	10	
3. What months is this?	10	
4. What is today's date?	10	
5. What day of the weak is this?	10	
6. What country are we in?	10	
7. Which state are we in?	10	
8. Which city/town are we in?	10	
9. In home—What is the street address of this house?	10	
10. In hospital—What is the name of this building	10	
II. **Registration** (Maximum score 3)		
SAY—I am going to name three objects, when I am finished, I want you to repeat them. Remember what they are because I am going to ask you to name them again in a few minutes. Say the following words slowly at 01 second interval ball/car/man. Give one point for each correct answer.	20	
III. **Attention and calculation** (Maximum score 5)	—	
Ask the client to begin at 100 and count backwards by 7. Stop after 5 subtractions (93, 86, 79, 72, 65). Give one point for each correct number or If the client cannot perform this task ask him/her to spell the word now spell it backwards. Give one point for each correctly placed letter.	3	
IV. **Recall** (Maximum score 3)	10	
Say what are the three objects I had asked you to remember		
V. **Language** (Maximum score 9)		
Naming	10	
– Show wrist watch. Ask what is this?		
– Show pencil. Ask what is this?	10	
Repetition	10	
– Say I would like you to repeat this phrase after me. No ifs, ands or buts.		
Three stage command	30	
– Give the subject a piece of blank paper and say. "Take the paper in your right hand fold it in half and put it on the floor. Give one point for each action performed correctly.		
Reading On a blank piece of paper print the sentence. "Close your eyes." SAY—read the words on the page and then do what it says. Score correctly only if he/she actually closes his/her eyes.	10	
Writing Hand the person a pencil and paper. SAY—write any complete sentence on the piece of paper (The sentence must make sense, ignore spelling errors).	30	

Contd...

Contd...

Components	Time Allowed (Seconds)	Score
Copying Place design, eraser and pencil in front of the person. SAY—copy this design please. Figure Allow multiple tries. Want until the person has finished and hands it back. All 10 angles need to be present and the two shapes must interest to score 1 point.	60	
Total		

Suggestions/Impression

_____
_____
_____
_____
_____
_____

INVESTIGATIONS IN PSYCHIATRY

The growing awareness of various physical conditions which can produce psychiatric symptoms and the increased use of biological therapies have made it mandatory that appropriate physical investigations should be carried out before starting any treatment and during it. They serve diagnostic, basal screening and monitoring purposes.

Routine Tests

- A complete hemogram (total and differential blood count, hemoglobin, ESR) and urinalysis are the basic minimum of routine test. Leucopenia and agranulocytosis are associated with certain medications. Treatment with lithium and neuroleptic malignant syndrome are often associated with leukocytosis.
- Fasting and post-prandial blood sugar, chest X-ray and an EEG are often considered routine tests.
- An EEG is necessary for monitoring cardiac effects of certain drugs.
- Serum electrolytes (sodium, potassium chlorides, bicarbonates, calcium, etc.) are sometimes needed as basal routine investigations. An electrolyte imbalance causes various neuropsychiatric symptoms like delirium.
- Liver function tests—serum glutamic oxaloacetic transaminase (SGOT), serum glutamic-pyruvic transaminase (SGPT), serum alkaline phosphatase, prothrombin time, serum bilirubin levels and serum proteins (total and differential) are some common liver function tests. Liver function tests are done for all alcoholic patients.
- Renal function tests—blood urea, serum creatinine and creatinine clearance, thyroid function tests (T3, T4 and TSH) and ECG are routinely done on patients prior to starting lithium therapy.
- Thyroid function test—usually done in refractory depression, rapid cycling mood disorder and treatment with lithium and carbamazepine.
- Drug levels—drug levels are indicated to test for therapeutic blood levels, for toxic blood levels and for testing drug compliance, e.g. lithium, carbamazepine, valproate, haloperidol, nortriptyline, imipramine, benzodiazepines, barbiturates.
- An ECG and chest X-ray are usually done before a patient is posted for ECT.

DIAGNOSTIC PROCEDURES USED TO DETECT ALTERED BRAIN FUNCTION

Several diagnostic procedures are used to detect alteration in biologic function that may contribute to psychiatric disorders.

1. Electroencephalography (EEG)

Technique: Electrodes are placed on the scalp in a standardized position. Amplitude and frequency of beta, alpha, theta and delta brain waves are graphically recorded on paper by ink markers for multiple areas of the brain surface.

Purpose: It measures brain electrical activity; identifies dysrhythmias, asymmetries, or suppression of brain rhythms; used in the diagnosis of epilepsy, neoplasm stroke, metabolic or degenerative disease.

2. Computed Tomography (CT)

Technique: Series of radiographs that are computer constructed into slices of the brain that can be stacked by the computer giving a three dimensional image.

Purpose: Measures accuracy of brain structure to detect possible lesion, abscesses, areas of infarction or aneurysm. CT has also identified various anatomic differences in clients, with schizophrenia, organic mental disorder and bipolar disorder.

3. Magnetic Resonance Imaging (MRI)

Technique: A magnetic field surrounding the head induces brain tissue to emit radio waves that are computerized to provide clear and detailed construction of sectional images of the brain. No radiation or contrast medium is used.

Purpose: Measures anatomic and biochemical status of various segments of the brain; detects brain edema, ischemia, infection, neoplasm, trauma and other changes such as demyelination. Morphological differences between the brains of clients with schizophrenia and those of control subjects have been noted.

4. Brain Electrical Activity Mapping (BEAM)

Technique: Uses computed tomographic techniques to display data derived from EEG recordings of brain electrical activity that can be sensory evoked by specific stimuli, such as flash of light or a sudden sound, or cognitive evoked by specific mental tasks.

Purpose: Measures brain electrical activity; used largely in research to represent statistical relationships between individuals and groups or between two populations of subject (e.g. client with schizophrenia vs. control subjects).

5. Positron Emission Tomography (PET)

Technique: An injected radioactive substance travels to the brain and shows up as a bright spot on the scan; different substances are taken up by the brain in different amounts, depending on the type of tissues and the level of activity.

Purpose: Measures specific brain functioning, such as glucose metabolism, oxygen utilization, blood flow, and of particular interest in psychiatry neurotransmitter/receptor interaction.

6. Single Photon Emission Computed Tomography (SPECT)

Technique: The technique is similar to PET but a longer acting radioactive substance must be used to allow time for a gamma camera to rotate about the head and gather the data, which are then assembled on the computer into a brain image.

Purpose: Measures various aspects of brain functioning as with PET; has also been used to image activity or cerebrospinal fluid circulation.

ASSIGNMENT 6: INVESTIGATIONS IN PSYCHIATRY

1. Write the nurses responsibility before and after the above stated diagnostic procedures.

2. Mention responsibilities of a nurse for any other/new diagnostic procedure that you observed during your posting

NEUROLOGICAL EXAMINATION

Neurological examination is done to determine the presence or absence of disease in the nervous system. Following are the aspects of neurological examination:

1. Levels of consciousness
2. Mental status examination
3. Special cerebral functions
4. Examination of the cranial nerves
5. Motor function
6. Sensory function
7. Cerebellar function
8. Reflexes

1. **Levels of consciousness:** It include the following areas for assessment:
   a. Alertness
   b. Lethargic
   c. Stuporous
   d. Semi-comatose
   e. Comatose.

A standardized method of measuring patient's level of consciousness is the Glasgow coma scale.

Glasgow Coma Scale

The Glasgow coma scale (GCS) is a numeric expression of cognition, behavior and neurologic function. It is the most commonly used scale and was designed to measure level of consciousness. It is based or the assessment of eye opening, verbal response and motor response. The total of the three scores ranges from 3 to 15, with 3 being the most severe and 15 being normal.

Glasgow coma scale

Best eye opening response	Spontaneously	4
	To speech	3
	To pain	2
	No response	1
Best motor response	Obeys verbal command	6
	Localizes pain	5
	Flekion—withdrawl	4
	Extension—abnormal	3
	No response	2
		1
Best verbal response	Orientation to time, place person	5
	Conversation confused	4
	Sounds incomprehensive	3
	No response	2
		1
Total score		15

2. **Mental status examination** (Refer page number 22)
3. **Special cerebral functions:**
   Assess for agnosia, apraxia and aphasia
   a. Agnosia—inability to recognize
      i. Common objects through senses.
   b. Apraxia—patient cannot carry out skilled act even in the absence of paralysis.
   c. Aphasia—inability to communicate.
4. **Examination of the cranial nerves:**
   When examining the cranial nerves one must be cognizant of asymmetry. The following is the summary of the Cranial Nerves and their respective functions as shown in Table 2.2.

Table 2.2: Functions of Cranial Nerves

Nerve		Function
Cranial nerve I (CN I)	Olfactory nerve	Smell
Cranial nerve (CN II)	Optic nerve	Visual acuity, visual fields, occular fundi
CN II + III	Optic + occulomotor nerve	Pupillary reaction
CN III, IV, VI	Occulomotor, Trochlear and Abducens nerve	Extraocular movements including opening of eyes
CN V	Trigeminal nerve	Facial sensations, movements of the jaw, and corneal reflexes
CN VII	Facial nerve	Facial movements and gustation
CN VIII	Acoustic nerve	Hearing and balance
CN IX, X	Glossopharyngeal and vagus nerve	Swallowing, elevation of the palate, gag reflex and gustation
CN V, VII, X, XII	Trigeminal, facial, Vagus, and hypoglossal nerve	Voice and speech
CN XI	Spinal accessory nerve	Shrugging the shoulders and turning of head
CN XII	Hypoglossal nerve	Movement and protrusion of tongue

5. **Motor function:**
   The motor function examination is divide into the following—body positioning, involuntary movements, muscle tone and muscle strength.
6. **Sensory function:**
   The sensory examination includes testing for pain sensation (pin prick), light touch sensation (brush), position sense, stereognosis, graphesthesia and extinction.
7. **Cerebellar function:**
   For evaluation of balance and coordination the following tests are used, e.g. Finger to finger test, Finger to nose test, Romberg's test and Tandom walking test.
8. **Reflex activity:**
   Reflex activity examination provides information about the nature, location and progression of neurological disorder.

Normal reflexes	Abnormal reflexes
1. Superficial reflex 　➢ Abdominal reflex 　➢ Plantar reflex 　➢ Corneal reflex 　➢ Pharangeal reflex 　➢ Cremasteric reflex 　➢ Anal reflex	➢ Babinski's sign ➢ Jaw reflex ➢ Palm-Chin 　− Clonus 　− Snout 　− Rooting 　− Sucking
2. Deep tendon reflex	Glabella ➢ Grasp ➢ Chewing

ASSIGNMENT 7: NEUROLOGICAL EXAMINATION

Q.1. List the equipments required for a neurological examination.

Q.2. Discuss in general nurses role in neurological examination.

Q.3. Perform a neurological examination.

PSYCHOLOGICAL ASSESSMENT

Psychological assessment can be used in pretreatment planning, assessing the progress of therapy and evaluating its effectiveness. Psychological tests may reveal considerable information concerning the patient's inner life, feelings and images that may facilitate therapy. Psychological assessment often needs the services of a clinical psychologist. The following is the list of instruments used for psychological assessment.

Instruments for Assessing Symptoms and Symptom Patterns

1. Brief psychiatric rating scale (BPRS)
2. Anxiety self-rating scale
3. Hamilton anxiety scale
4. Beck's depression inventory (BDI)
5. Hamilton depression scale (HAMD)
6. Manic state rating scale
7. Nurses observation scale for inpatient evaluation (NOSIE)
8. Positive and negative symptom scale (PANSS) for schizophrenia
9. Scale for assessment of positive symptoms (SAPS)
10. Scale for assessment of negative symptoms (SANS)
11. The CAGE questionnaire
12. Mini mental state examination (MMSE).

Instruments for Assessment of Personality Traits and Disorders

1. Minnesota multiphasic personality inventory (MMPI)
2. Cattell's 16 Factor personality inventory.

Instruments for Assessment of Cognitive Functioning

1. Wechsler adult intelligence scale (WAIS)
2. Wechsler intelligence scale for children (WISC)
3. Raven's standard progressive matrices
4. Raven's coloured progressive matrices
5. Bhatia battery test of intelligence
6. Bender gestalt test.

Instruments for Assessment of Psychodynamics

1. Rorschach Inkblot test
2. Thematic apperception test
3. Sentence completion test.

Instruments for Assessment of Environmental Stressors

1. Social adjustment scale
2. Marital satisfaction inventory.

ASSIGNMENT 8: PSYCHOLOGICAL TESTS

1. Write in brief about any three instruments used for psychological assessment.
   (Note: Each instrument should belong to different category).

3. The Nursing Process

OVERVIEW

The nursing process provides a methodology by which nurses may deliver care using a systematic, scientific approach. The focus is goal directed and based on a decision-making or problem solving model, consisting of six steps—assessment, diagnosis, outcome identification, planning, implementation and evaluation.

Nursing process is dynamic, not static. It is an ongoing process that continues for as long as the nurse and client have interactions directed towards change in the client's physical or behavioral response. Figure 3.1 presents a schematic diagram of the ongoing nursing process.

I. ASSESSMENT

The psychiatric-mental health nurse collects client health data. Information for this database is gathered from a variety of sources including interview with the client or family, observing the client and his or her environment, consulting other health team members, reviewing the client's records and conducting a nursing physical examination.

II. DIAGNOSIS

In the second step, data gathered during the assessment are analyzed. Diagnosis and potential problem statements are formulated and prioritized. Diagnosis conform to accepted classification systems such as the NANDA nursing diagnosis classification.

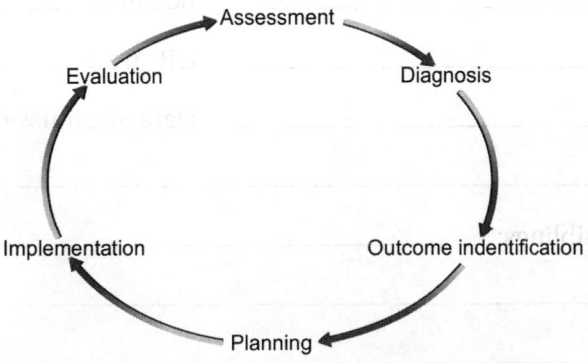

Fig. 3.1: The ongoing nursing process

III. OUTCOME IDENTIFICATION

The P/MHN (Psychiatric/mental health nurse) identifies expected outcomes—individualized to the client. Expected outcomes are derived from the diagnosis. They must be measurable and estimate a time for attainment. They must be realistic for the client's capabilities and are most effective when formulated by the team members, the client and significant others together.

IV. PLANNING

The P/MHN develops a plan of care that prescribes interventions to attain expected outcomes. The care plan is individualized to the client's mental health problems, conditions or needs and is developed in collaboration with client, significant others and team members. For each diagnosis identified, the most appropriate interventions, based on current psychiatric/mental health nursing practice and research, are selected. Client education and necessary referrals are included. Priorities for delivery of nursing care are determined.

V. IMPLEMENTATION

The P/MHN implements the interventions identified in the plan of care. She uses a wide range of interventions designed to prevent mental and physical illness and promote, maintain and restore mental and physical health. Documentation of interventions also occurs at this step in the nursing process.

VI. EVALUATION

The P/MHN evaluates the client's progress in attaining expected outcomes. The client's responses to treatment is documented, validating use of the nursing process in the delivery for care. The diagnosis, outcomes and plan of care are reviewed and revised as need is determined by the evaluation.

ASSIGNMENT 9: NURSING PROCESS/CARE PLAN

Identification data

Name: _____ Ward: _____

Age: _____ Bed no.: _____

Sex: _____ CR no.: _____

Father/husband name: _____ Date of admission: _____

Marital status: _____

Number and ages of children/siblings: _____

Spouse/parents age: _____

Living arrangements: _____

Occupation: _____

Education: _____

Religion: _____ Nationality: _____

Mother tongue: _____

Address: _____

Brought by/informant: _____

Diagnosis/provisional diagnosis: _____

Brief History of Patient's illness

_____
_____
_____
_____
_____
_____
_____
_____
_____
_____
_____
_____
_____
_____
_____
_____
_____
_____
_____
_____
_____

Mental status examination

DAY – I

Assessment	Nursing Diagnosis	Goals
Subjective data:		
Objective data:		

Planning	Implementation	Evaluation

DAY – II

Assessment	Nursing Diagnosis	Goals
Subjective data:		
Objective data:		

Planning	Implementation	Evaluation

DAY – III

Assessment	Nursing Diagnosis	Goals
Subjective data:		
Objective data:		

Planning	Implementation	Evaluation

DAY – IV

Assessment	Nursing Diagnosis	Goals
Subjective data:		
Objective data:		

Planning	Implementation	Evaluation

DAY – V

Assessment	Nursing Diagnosis	Goals
Subjective data:		
Objective data:		

Planning	Implementation	Evaluation

SUMMARY

4 | Communication Techniques

OVERVIEW

Communication is basic to all human performance and interaction. All communication must be aimed at preserving the self respect of both individuals. Although seemingly simple on the surface, these techniques are difficult and require practice. If they are used appropriately they can enhance the nurses effectiveness to patient care. Hays and Larsen (1963) have identified a number of techniques to assist the nurse in interacting more therapeutically with patients.

THERAPEUTIC COMMUNICATION TECHNIQUES

1. Using silence
2. Accepting
3. Giving recognition
4. Offering self
5. Giving board openings
6. Offering general leads
7. Placing the event in time or sequence
8. Making observation
9. Encouraging description of perceptions
10. Encouraging comparison
11. Restating
12. Reflecting
13. Focusing
14. Exploring
15. Seeking clarification and validation
16. Presenting reality
17. Voicing doubt
18. Verbalizing the implied
19. Attempting to translate feelings into words
20. Formulating a plan of action.

NON-THERAPEUTIC COMMUNICATION TECHNIQUES

1. Giving reassurance
2. Rejecting
3. Giving approval or disapproval
4. Agreeing/disagreeing
5. Giving advice
6. Probing
7. Defending
8. Requesting an explanation
9. Indicating the existence of an external source of power
10. Belittling feelings expressed
11. Making Stereotyped comments
12. Using dental
13. Interpreting
14. Introducing an unrelated topic.

NONVERBAL BEHAVIORS FOR ATTENTIVE LISTENING

S— Sit squarely facing the person
O— Observe an open posture
L— Lean forward toward the patient
E— Establish eye contact
R— Relax.

HOW TO DEVELOP LISTENING SKILLS

Good Listeners Make Good Communicators

1. Stop talking sometimes
2. Put the audience at ease
3. Concentrate on what someone is saying
4. Ensure you are not distracted
5. Avoid making assumptions
6. Look for hidden or deeper messages
7. Ask questions
8. Listen actively; restate and rephrase.

PROCESS RECORDING

Overview

Travelbee (1979) defined process recording as a systematic method of collecting data prior to interpreting, analyzing and synthesizing the data obtained.

Process recordings are written reports of verbal interaction with clients. They are verbatim accounts written by the learner/nurses as a tool for improving interpersonal communication techniques. The process recording can take many forms but usually includes verbal and nonverbal communication of both nurse and client. The process recording is not documentation in and of itself but should be used as a learning tool for professional development.

The purpose of process recording is to improve the quality of patient care and simultaneously that of the learning experience, as it encourages the learner to attend to what is happening. In addition, process recording facilitates the Integration of theory and practice; increased self awareness through the identification of thoughts and feelings, verbal and nonverbal communication, development of learner's observational skills; competence in collection, analysis and synthesis of data; development of learner's ability to identify nursing problems and competencies necessary to solve them.

Stages of Process Recording

A brief description of each of the stages will be given here, a more detailed account can be found in Travelbee (1979).

Stage 1: Collection of Raw Data

The nurse has a responsibility to inform the patient during her first interaction with him. This stage includes the verbal and nonverbal communication of both the learner and patient during the interaction.

Stage 2: Interpretation

This is one of the most difficult phases for the learner. Here she must be able to explain that which is not explicit, to comprehend the probable meaning of data and recognize the relevance to nursing. This takes place after the interaction has been completed and can be at different levels ranging from assumption to hypothesis.

Stage 3: Application of Concepts

In order to be able to apply concepts, the nurse must process an understanding of the body of knowledge underlying nursing practice, that is, the principles and concepts used to explain and predict behavior in nursing situations.

Stage 4: Analysis

This involves separating the data into component parts in order to critically assess its nature and significance. It is important to look at each part and its relationship to the whole.

Stage 5: Synthesis

This is concerned with the process of putting the analyzed parts of the data together to form a complete whole. It is as a result of the analysis and synthesis that the learner is able to plan future interactions.

Items to be Included in the Process Recording

1. Date, time, place and duration of the interaction.
2. The learner's thoughts and feelings prior to the interaction.

3. Objectives for the interaction—these are the statements of the goals for the interaction.
4. The interaction will include as much as possible of the communication, both verbal and nonverbal, as well as any periods of silence.
5. Learner's thoughts and feelings following the interaction.
6. Evaluation of the interaction: This will be assessed in terms of how well the objectives for the intervention were achieved.
7. Planning for the next interaction.
8. Identification of the customary pattern of reacting. It is important for the learner to examine her own behavior and identify her strengths and weaknesses.

ASSIGNMENT 10: PROCESS RECORDING

1. Identification data

Name: _____ Ward: _____

Age: _____ Bed no.: _____

Sex: _____ CR no.: _____

Father/husband name: _____ Date of admission: _____

Marital status: _____

Number and ages of children/siblings: _____

Spouse/parents age: _____

Living arrangements: _____

Occupation: _____

Education: _____

Religion: _____ Nationality: _____

Mother tongue: _____

Address: _____

Brought by/informant: _____

Diagnosis/provisional diagnosis: _____

2. Presenting complaints _____
_____
_____

Communication Techniques

3. History of present illness

4. Objectives of interview

Interview: I

Day—I _____

Date _____

Time _____

Venue _____

Specific objectives _____

_____

_____

_____

_____

_____

_____

_____

Participants	Conversation	Communication Technique	Inference

Communication Techniques

Participants	Conversation	Communication Technique	Inference

Participants	Conversation	Communication Technique	Inference

Communication Techniques

Participants	Conversation	Communication Technique	Inference

Participants	Conversation	Communication Technique	Inference

Summary

_____
_____
_____
_____
_____
_____
_____
_____
_____
_____

Introspection

Interview: II

Day—2

Date

Time

Venue

Specific objectives

Participants	Conversation	Communication Technique	Inference

Participants	Conversation	Communication Technique	Inference

Participants	Conversation	Communication Technique	Inference

Communication Techniques

Participants	Conversation	Communication Technique	Inference

Participants	Conversation	Communication Technique	Inference

Communication Techniques

Summary

_____
_____
_____
_____
_____
_____
_____
_____
_____
_____
_____
_____
_____

Introspection

Interview III

Day—3 _____

Date _____

Time _____

Venue _____

Specific objectives _____

_____
_____
_____
_____
_____
_____
_____
_____

Participants	Conversation	Communication Technique	Inference

Participants	Conversation	Communication Technique	Inference

Participants	Conversation	Communication Technique	Inference

Communication Techniques

Participants	Conversation	Communication Technique	Inference

Participants	Conversation	Communication Technique	Inference

Summary

Introspection

Interview: IV

Day—4

Date

Time

Venue

Specific objectives

Participants	Conversation	Communication Technique	Inference

Participants	Conversation	Communication Technique	Inference

Participants	Conversation	Communication Technique	Inference

Communication Techniques

Participants	Conversation	Communication Technique	Inference

Participants	Conversation	Communication Technique	Inference

Summary

Introspection

Interview: V

Day—6

Date

Time

Venue

Specific objectives

Participants	Conversation	Communication Technique	Inference

Communication Techniques

Participants	Conversation	Communication Technique	Inference

Participants	Conversation	Communication Technique	Inference

Communication Techniques

Participants	Conversation	Communication Technique	Inference

Participants	Conversation	Communication Technique	Inference

Summary

Introspection

Total summary

Introspection

Learning experience and evaluation

5 Case Presentation

ASSIGNMENT 11: CASE PRESENTATION

1. Identification data

Name: _____ Ward: _____

Age: _____ Bed no.: _____

Sex: _____ CR no.: _____

Father/husband name: _____ Date of admission: _____

Marital status: _____

Number and ages of children/siblings: _____

Spouse/parents age: _____

Living arrangements: _____

Occupation: _____

Education: _____

Religion: _____ Nationality: _____

Mother tongue: _____

Address: _____

Brought by/informant: _____

Diagnosis/provisional diagnosis: _____

Brief history of patient: _____

_____

_____

Brief history of Patient's illness

Mental status examination

LESSON PLAN OF CASE PRESENTATION ON _____

Group: _____

Size of group: _____

Venue: _____

Date: _____

Time: _____

Previous knowledge: _____

Methods of teaching: _____

AV Aids: _____

General objectives: _____

Time	Specific Objectives	Content

Case Presentation

Teaching learning activity	AV Aids	Evaluation

Time	Specific Objectives	Content

Case Presentation

Teaching learning activity	AV Aids	Evaluation

Time	Specific Objectives	Content

Case Presentation

Teaching learning activity	AV Aids	Evaluation

Time	Specific Objectives	Content

Case Presentation

Teaching learning activity	AV Aids	Evaluation

Summary

Bibliography

6 | Therapeutic Modalities

ELECTROCONVULSIVE THERAPY

Overview

Electroconvulsive therapy (ECT) is a treatment in which a grand mal seizure is artificially induced through the application of an electric current to the brain while client is under general anesthesia. The current is applied through electrodes placed bilaterally on the frontal temporal region or unilaterally on the same side as the dominant hand. Most clients require six to ten treatments.

History

The first electroconvulsive therapy was performed in 1938 in Rome by Italian psychiatrists Ugo Cerlette and Lucio Bini. Electroconvulsive therapy was widely accepted from around 1940–1955. This period was followed by a 20 years span during which ECT was considered objectionable. A second peak of acceptance began around 1975 and has been increasing to the present.

Procedure

Electroconvulsive therapy involves the passage of an electrical stimulus of 70–150 volts to the brain for 0.7–1.5 seconds to produce a grand mal seizure. Seizure induction is necessary to achieve the therapeutic effect, which is thought to be the result of an alteration in the postsynaptic response to the neurotransmitters in the central nervous system.

The client receives atropine sulfate subcutaneously before the procedure and at the beginning of the treatment an intravenous dose of sodium pentothal. Electrode jelly is applied bilaterally to the temples or unilaterally to the padded electrodes. An airway or soft mouth gag is put in the client's mouth to prevent tongue bite. Succinyl choline is also administered. The resulting grand mal seizure closely resembles a tonic phase (tightening of muscles) for approximately 10 seconds and a clonic phase (rhythmic movements of the muscles) for 30 seconds. The movements are slight and often limited to plantar flexion of the feet, followed by rhythmic twitching of the toes. The seizure is accompanied by a short period of apnea and then stertorous (snoring like) respiration. Because the muscle relaxant paralyses the respiratory muscles an anesthetist is present to administer oxygen to the client and assist respiration by mechanical means if necessary. Usually, the client sleeps for 5–10 minutes after seizure, slowly awakens and does not remember the treatment.

Indications

- Treatment of intractable depression, that is severe depression in which antidepressant medications have been ineffective or not tolerated well.
- Treatment of manic episodes of bipolar disorders whereby therapy with lithium or other medications are ineffective or not tolerated well.
- Shown to induce remission with clients who present with acute schizophrenia, but is of little value to treat chronic schizophrenia.
- Catatonia responds well to ECT with improvement in motor symptoms (posturing, rigidity, catalepsy).

Contraindications

There are no absolute contraindications to ECT, however, relative contraindications are—
- Increased intracranial pressure
- Cerebrovascular accident
- Space occupying intracranial lesions
- Cervical injury or problem
- Head injuries
- Recent myocardial infarction.

Types

1. Modified—treatment approach whereby pretreatment medications are utilized to initiate treatment.
2. Unmodified—treatment without the aid of medication. A concern with this approach is the high morbidity associated with treatment, thus, this method is no longer in use.

Risks Associated with ECT

1. Mortality—death is rare and usually is related to cardiovascular complications.
2. Cognitive impairment memory loss has both retrograde and anterograde components.
3. Brain damage.

ASSIGNMENT 12: ELECTROCONVULSIVE THERAPY

1. Describe and draw the physical layout of an ECT room.

_____
_____
_____
_____
_____

2. List the equipment required for electroconvulsive therapy.

3. What are the medications used in ECT.

a.

b.

c.

4. Describe pretreatment nursing care.

5. Describe nursing care during the procedure.

6. Describe post-treatment nursing care.

Therapeutic Modalities

7. Complete the following record for two of your patients you assisted during ECT.

CASE NO. 1

Identification data

Name : _____ CR no.: _____

Age/sex : _____ Bed no.: _____

Date : _____ Ward: _____

Diagnosis : _____

Number of ECT received : _____

Time	Vital signs				
Before the procedure	Temperature	Pulse	Respiration	Blood Pressure	Level of consciousness

After the procedure

Any other observation:

_____

_____

_____

_____

_____

_____

_____

_____

CASE NO. 2

Identification data

Name : _____ CR no.: _____

Age/sex : _____ Bed no.: _____

Date : _____ Ward : _____

Diagnosis : _____

Number of ECT received : _____

Time	Vital signs				
Before the procedure	Temperature	Pulse	Respiration	Blood pressure	Level of consciousness

After the procedure

Any other observation:

_____

_____

_____

_____

_____

_____

_____

_____

RESTRAINING

Overview

Psychiatric facilities often use medical interventions in the form of restraints to reduce safety risk posed by voilent patients and to prevents patients from harming self and others. The term restraint includes either physical restraint or a drug that is being used as a restraint. A physical restraint is any manual method or physical or mechanical device, maternal or equipment attached or adjacent to the patient's body that he or she cannot easily remove, that restricts freedom of movement or normal access to one's body. A drug used as a restraint is a medication used to control behavior or to restrict the patient's freedom of movement and is not a standard treatment for the patient's medical or psychiatric conditions.

1. **Chemical Restraints:** If agitation continues to escalate inspite of attemtps to defuse the enger beginning with the least restrictive means, offer client choice of taking medication voluntarily. If he or she refuses reassess the situation to determine if harm to self or others is imminent. Chemical restraints are medications used to restrict the patient's freedom of movement or for emergency control of behavior but are not a standard treatment for the patient's medical or psychiatric condition.

2. **Physical Restraints:** Physical restraints manually leather straps, bed sheet or bandages, immobilize the patient who cannot control aggressive impulses and who is potentially dangerous to himself or others. Behaviors considered clinically justified for restrains are the following:
   a. Accelerated motor activity
   b. Physical assault to self others and environment
   c. Physical and verbal threats
   d. Hyper-responsiveness to environmental stimuli.

Restraints should not be used as punishment or retaliation or to free staff members from having to observe or client. Continuous supervision is necessary during restraint to prevent untoward effects such as suffocation or injury to an extremity. Restraints are applied only in a horizontal line that is to both hands and both feet. Cross restraints (one arm and the opposite leg or one arm and one leg on the same side) are extremely dangerous and unacceptable. Also improper use of restraints can lead to patient harm and potential civil litigation.

Seclusion: Seclusion confines a client to a single room. The door may be locked or unlocked. There may be minimal furnishings and a limited opportunity for communication with others. It is an appropriate method for controlling behavior, especially when a client has been destructive to the physical environment, is hyperactive or has been extremely agitated by environmental stimuli. Seclusion is not indicated for clients who are actively suicidal when a client is put in seclusion, the procedure is carried out as that for the restrained client. A seclusion register should be maintained and the fifteen minutes nursing observation should be fully documented.

Seclusion and mechanical restraints have now largely been eliminated from the repertoire of mental health case. However, there is still very small number of instances when these measures are resorted to but this should only happen as a last resort.

ASSIGNMENT 13: RESTRAINING

Q.1. Write the nursing interventions related to physical/chemical restraints, that you might have assisted or applied to a patient in the ward.

Q.2. Document the incident precipitating a client's seclusion and records the client's response, length of seclusion, and all the nursing care given during seclusion.

PSYCHOPHARMACOTHERAPY

Overview

Psychopharmacologic agents (also called psychotropic or psychotherapeutic medications) are able to relieve symptoms, but not "cure mental illness." Clients taking psychotropic medications and their families need education regarding the medications action, purpose, intended effects, side effects, toxic or dangerous effects, treatment for side-effects and what to do about adverse or toxic effects. Non-adherence must be managed; client may not remember to take psychotropic medications or may refuse to take them at all or as prescribed. Medications may need to be changed and/or dosage adjusted in accordance with drug effectiveness and client response. Nurses must observe and document the client's responses to and beliefs about medications.

Principles of Psychopharmacotherapy

- Psychopharmacologic agents do not "cure" mental illness.
- Clients require physical and psychiatric assessments before psychotropic medication is prescribed for them.
- Clients hold various views about the use of psychotropic medications; some of these views may bring about nonadherence to medication treatment.
- Clients must give informed consent prior to administration of psychotropic medication including an explanation of risks versus benefits.
- Psychotropic medication have different onsets of actions. Most medications (Lithium, antidepressants) require daily administration for one to several weeks before their intended effects are evident; some medications (benzodiazepines, antipsychotics) act more immediately.

Purposes of Psychotropic Medications

- Relieve or reduce symptoms of dysfunctional thoughts, moods, or actions, mental illness or disorder.
- Improve client's functioning
- Increase client's adherence (or compliance) and amenability to other therapies.
- Most psychotropic medications act by modulating neurotransmitters (brain chemicals), specifically serotonin norepinephrine (noradrenaline), dopamine, acetylcholine and glutamate.

Reasons for Noncompliance to Psychotropic Medication Regimen

- Medications may be expensive and the client cannot afford them.
- Clients may refuse to take medications because of their unpleasant or distressing side-effects.
- Clients may stop taking their medications because they begin to feel better and believe that they no longer need the medications.
- Clients may not believe they have any illness requiring medication or fear the stigma associated with having a mental illness and taking medication.
- Mental illness itself such as paranoia, contributes to the client's denial or fears about medication usage.

Services that Encourage Adherence to Medication Regimen

➢ Follow up interactions with the client will help the nurse verify that the client understands the purpose, proper administration, intended effects, side and toxic effects of, and how to treat serious problems associated with psychotropic medications.
➢ Support persons can encourage and assist the client's adherence to his or her psychotropic medication regimen.
➢ Appropriate laboratory tests must be conducted to prevent serious complications and assure safe and therapeutic level of psychotropic medication.
➢ Medication groups often provide not only education, but also peer support to those taking psychotropic medication. Often clients and their families have misconceptions that are preventing the client from taking his or her medication.
➢ Depot injections (injections of medication into a body area where it will be deposited and stored) of antipsychotic medication can provide two to four weeks dosage of the medication to clients who have difficulty adhering to their medication schedule.

Effect on Special Populations

Children

Psychotropic medications should be administered with great caution to children. Initiating treatment with small dosages and increasing the dosages slowly diminishes the likelihood of side effects. Although the small volume of distribution suggests the use of lower doses than in adults, a child's higher rate of metabolism suggest that a higher ratio of mg of drug to kg of body weight should be used.

Elderly

➢ Elderly clients are more susceptible to side effects, especially cardiac effects and may metabolize and excrete drugs more slowly.
➢ Lower doses are needed for the elderly client because of decreased liver and renal function.
➢ Elderly clients are likely to be taking other drugs; therefore, they have an increased risk for drug-drug interactions.
➢ They may have decreased liver and renal function, therefore, their BUN (Blood, Urea, Nitrogen), creatinine and liver enzymes should be monitored regularly.
➢ Regular use of sedating medications for sleep should be discouraged because they usually return to normal sleeping patterns after only a few nights of medication use.
➢ Discourage sedating medications as they may cause excessive sedation, confusion or disorientation resulting in falls and other injuries.

Pregnancy

The basic rule is to avoid administering any drug to a woman who is pregnant (particularly during the first trimester) or who is breastfeeding a child. This rule however, occasionally needs to be broken when the mother's psychiatric disorder is severe.

BASIC PHARMACOLOGIC PRINCIPLES

- **Pharmacokinetics:** It refers to the movement of medication molecules in the body, including absorption, distribution, metabolism and excretion of medications.
- **Absorption:** The movement of a medication from its site of administration (e.g. GI tract, muscle, skin or subcutaneous tissue) tissue to the blood stream.
- **Distribution:** The transportation of a medication to its site of action by bodily fluids.
- **Metabolism:** Occurs primarily in the liver. Individuals diagnosed with liver dysfunction have a decreased ability to metabolize medications and are at risk of undue accumulation of medication and possible toxicity.
- **Excretion:** The elimination of a medication from the body primarily through the kidneys. Individuals diagnosed with renal dysfunction should be monitored for an increase in duration and intensity of medication responses.
- **Medication Responses:** Plasma medication levels can be regulated to control medication responses. Medication dosing attempts to maintain plasma levels between the minimum effective concentration (MEC) and the toxic concentration. When a medication has achieved plasma levels that are effective and not toxic, the plasma level is within the therapeutic range.
- **Therapeutic Index (TI):** Medications with a high TI have a wide safety margin. Therefore, there is no need for routine serum medication level monitoring. Medications with a low TI should have serum medication level monitored closely. Monitor peak levels based on the route of administration. For example, an oral medication may have a peak of 1 to 3 hours after administration. Whereas if the medication is given intravenously, the peak time might occur within 10 minutes.
- **Half Life:** The plasma half life is the time taken for the plasma concentration of the drug to decline to one-half of its value.
- **Pharmacodynamics:** (Mechanism of action) Describes the interactions between medications and target cell, body systems, and organs to produce effects. Medications interact with cells in one or two ways. Medications can mimic the receptor activity regulated by endogenous compounds or block normal receptor activity regulated by endogenous compounds. For example, morphine is classified as an agonist because it activates the receptors that produce analgesia sedation, constipation, and other effects.

KEY POINTS/KNOWLEDGE REQUIRED PRIOR TO MEDICATION ADMINISTRATION

Medication category/class: Medications may be organized according to pharmacologic action, therapeutic use, body system, chemical make up, and safe use during pregnancy.
Mechanism of action: This is how the medication produces the desired therapeutic effect.
Therapeutic effect: This is the primary action for which the medication is administered to a specific client.
Adverse effects: These are any unintended or undesired effect that can occur at a normal medication dose.
Side effects: These are secondary medication effects that occur at therapeutic doses. These are usually predictable.
Drug-drug interaction: Some medications may be given together to increase or decrease the therapeutic effect. Two medications together may increase or decrease the adverse side effects.

Drug food interaction: Food may alter medication absorption and/or may contain substances that react with certain medications.

Toxicity: An adverse medication effect that is considered severe and may be life-threatening. It can be caused by an excessive dose, but can occur at therapeutic dose levels.

Contraindication/precautions:
- A specific medication can be contraindicated for a client based on the client's condition. For example, a patient with history of allergy to a particular medication.
- Precautions should be taken for a client who is more likely to have an adverse reaction than another client. For example, morphine depresses respiratory function, so it should be used with caution for clients who have impaired respiratory function.

Preparation, dosage and administration: It is important to know any special considerations for preparation, recommended doses and how to administer the medication.

Nursing implications: Know how to monitor therapeutic effects prevent and treat adverse effects provide for comfort, and instruct clients in the safe use of medications.

SAFE MEDICATION ADMINISTRATION: THE SEVEN RIGHTS

- **Right client:** Verify the client's identification each time a medication is given check identification band, name and/or photograph.
- **Right drug:** Correctly interpret medication order (verify completeness and clarity); read label three times; when container is selected, when removing dose from container, and when container is replaced; leave unit dose medication in its package until administration.
- **Right dose:** Calculate correct medication dose; check drug reference to ensure dose is within usual range.
- **Right time:** Give medication on time to maintain consistent therapeutic blood level. It is generally acceptable to give the medication half an hour before or after the scheduled time.
- **Right route:** Select the correct preparation for the ordered route. Know how to safely and correctly administer medication.
- **Right documentation:** Immediately records pertinent information, including client's responses to the medication.
- **Right to refuse:** Clients have the right to refuse to take a medication. Determine the reason for refusal, provide information regarding risk for refusal, notify appropriate health care personnel and document refusal and action taken.

PSYCHOPHARMACOLOGIC DRUGS

Category	Subcategory
1. Anxiolytics	– Benzodiazepine – Non-benzodiazepine
2. Antipsychotics	– Typical – Atypical
3. Antidepressants	– Selective serotonin reuptake inhibitor (SSRI) – Serotonin norepinephrine reuptake inhibitor (SNRI) – Norepinephrine dopamine reuptake inhibitor (NDRI) – Alpha 2 antagonist (NaSSA) – Serotonin 2 antagonist reuptake inhibitor (SARI) – Tricyclics (TCA) – Tetracyclics – Monoamine oxidase inhibitors (MAOI)
4. Mood stabilizers	– Antimanic (lithium) – Anticonvulsants
5. Psychostimulants (sympathomimetics)	– Methylphenidate – Combination or amphetamine salts – Dextroamphetamine
6. Sedative-hypnotic	– Barbiturates – Benzodiazepines – Benzodiazepines-like
7. Antiparkinsonian agents	– Anticholinergics – Antihistamines – Dopamine agonists
8. Deaddiction agents	– Treatment of opioid dependence – Treatment for alcohol – Treatment for nicotine
9. Any other	

ASSIGNMENT 14: PSYCHOPHARMACOLOGY

Category: Anxiolytics

Subcategory: Benzodiazepine

Commonly used drugs:

Action:

Intended effects:

Side or adverse effects:

Contraindications:

Nurses responsibility/unique teaching need/client education:

Therapeutic Modalities

Subcategory: Non-Benzodiazepine

Commonly used drugs:

Action:

Intended effects:

Side or adverse effects:

Contraindications:

Nurses responsibility/unique teaching need/client education:

Therapeutic Modalities

Category: Antipsychotics
Subcategory: Typical
Commonly used drugs:

Action:

Intended effects:

Side or adverse effects:

Contraindications:

Nurses responsibility/unique teaching need/client education:

Subcategory: Atypical
Commonly used drugs:

Action:

Intended effects:

Side or adverse effects:

Contraindications:

Nurses responsibility/unique teaching need/client education:

Therapeutic Modalities

Category: Antidepressants

Subcategory: Selective serotonin reuptake inhibitor (SSRI)

Commonly used drugs:

Action:

Intended effects:

Side or adverse effects:

Contraindications:

Nurses responsibility/unique teaching need/client education:

Subcategory: Serotonin norepinephrine reuptake inhibitor (SNRI)
Commonly used drugs:

Action:

Intended effects:

Side or adverse effects:

Contraindications:

Nurses responsibility/unique teaching need/client education:

Subcategory: Norepinephrine dopamine reuptake inhibitor (NDRI)
Commonly used drugs:

Action:

Intended effects:

Side or adverse effects:

Contraindications:

Nurses responsibility/unique teaching need/client education:

Therapeutic Modalities

Subcategory: Alpha 2 antagonist (NaSSA)

Commonly used drugs:

Action:

Intended effects:

Side or adverse effects:

Contraindications:

Nurses responsibility/unique teaching need/client education:

Therapeutic Modalities

Subcategory: Serotonin 2 antagonist reuptake inhibitor (SARI)

Commonly used drugs:
___

Action:
___

Intended effects:
___

Side or adverse effects:
___

Contraindications:
___

Nurses responsibility/unique teaching need/client education:

Subcategory: Tricyclics (TCA)
Commonly used drugs:
___

Action:
___

Intended effects:
___

Side or adverse effects:
___

Contraindications:
___

Nurses responsibility/unique teaching need/client education:

Therapeutic Modalities

Subcategory: Tetracyclics

Commonly used drugs:

Action:

Intended effects:

Side or adverse effects:

Contraindications:

Nurses responsibility/unique teaching need/client education:

Therapeutic Modalities

Subcategory: Monoamine oxidase inhibitors (MAOI)

Commonly used drugs:
____

Action:
____

Intended effects:
____

Side or adverse effects:
____

Contraindications:
____

Nurses responsibility/unique teaching need/client education:

Therapeutic Modalities

Category: Mood stabilizers
Subcategory: Antimanic (lithium)
Commonly used drugs:
___

Action:
___

Intended effects:
___

Side or adverse effects:
___

Contraindications:
___

Nurses responsibility/unique teaching need/client education:

Subcategory: Anticonvulsants
Commonly used drugs:
_____
_____
_____
_____
_____

Action:
_____
_____
_____
_____
_____

Intended effects:
_____
_____
_____
_____
_____

Side or adverse effects:
_____
_____
_____
_____

Contraindications:
_____
_____
_____
_____

Nurses responsibility/unique teaching need/client education:

Category: Psychostimulants (sympathomimetics)
Subcategory: Methylphenidate

Commonly used drugs:

Action:

Intended effects:

Side or adverse effects:

Contraindications:

Nurses responsibility/unique teaching need/client education:

Therapeutic Modalities

Subcategory: Combination or amphetamine salts

Commonly used drugs:
___

Action:
___

Intended effects:
___

Side or adverse effects:
___

Contraindications:
___

Nurses responsibility/unique teaching need/client education:

Subcategory: Dextroamphetamine
Commonly used drugs:

Action:

Intended effects:

Side or adverse effects:

Contraindications:

Nurses responsibility/unique teaching need/client education:

Therapeutic Modalities

Category: Sedative-hypnotic
Subcategory: Barbiturates
Commonly used drugs:

Action:

Intended effects:

Side or adverse effects:

Contraindications:

Nurses responsibility/unique teaching need/client education:

Therapeutic Modalities

Subcategory: Benzodiazepines

Commonly used drugs:

Action:

Intended effects:

Side or adverse effects:

Contraindications:

Nurses responsibility/unique teaching need/client education:

Therapeutic Modalities 177

Subcategory: Benzodiazepines-like
Commonly used drugs:

Action:

Intended effects:

Side or adverse effects:

Contraindications:

Nurses responsibility/unique teaching need/client education:

Category: Antiparkinsonian agent
Subcategory: Anticholinergics
Commonly used drugs:

Action:

Intended effects:

Side or adverse effects:

Contraindications:

Nurses responsibility/unique teaching need/client education:

Subcategory: Antihistamines

Commonly used drugs:

Action:

Intended effects:

Side or adverse effects:

Contraindications:

Nurses responsibility/unique teaching need/client education:

Subcategory: Dopamine agonists

Commonly used drugs:

Action:

Intended effects:

Side or adverse effects:

Contraindications:

Nurses responsibility/unique teaching need/client education:

Therapeutic Modalities

Category: Deaddiction Agents
Subcategory: Treatment of opioid dependence
Commonly used drugs:

Action:

Intended effects:

Side or adverse effects:

Contraindications:

Nurses responsibility/unique teaching need/client education:

Subcategory: Treatment for alcohol
Commonly used drugs:

Action:

Intended effects:

Side or adverse effects:

Contraindications:

Nurses responsibility/unique teaching need/client education:

Subcategory: Treatment for nicotine

Commonly used drugs:

Action:

Intended effects:

Side or adverse effects:

Contraindications:

Nurses responsibility/unique teaching need/client education:

Category: Any other

Commonly used drugs:

Action:

Intended effects:

Side or adverse effects:

Contraindications:

Nurses responsibility/unique teaching need/client education:

ASSIGNMENT 15: DRUG PRESENTATION

Conduct a drug presentation on any one drug: _____

Topic: _____

Group: _____

Size of group: _____

Venue: _____

Date: _____

Time: _____

Previous knowledge: _____

Method of teaching: _____

AV aids: _____

General objectives: _____

_____

_____

_____

_____

_____

_____

_____

_____

_____

_____

_____

_____

_____

_____

_____

Time	Specific Objectives	Content

Therapeutic Modalities

Teaching learning activity	AV Aids	Evaluation

Time	Specific Objectives	Content

Therapeutic Modalities

Teaching learning activity	AV Aids	Evaluation

Summary

Bibliography

PSYCHOSOCIAL THERAPIES

Behavior Therapy

Overview

Behavior is the internal and external response (feelings, thoughts, words, actions and physiological responses), a person makes to environmental stimuli. Behaviors are measurable and able to be altered through behavior therapy. Behavior and cognitive therapy is based on the concept that mental disorder represent learned behavior. Learning principles are applied to modify these behaviors. Behavioral techniques include the use of token economies, time out, and rewards or reinforcement for desired behaviors.

Types of Behavior Therapy

Classical Conditioning

If an unconditioned stimulus (food) elicits an unconditioned response (salivation in a hungry dog), then a conditioned stimulus (a bell) paired with food, over time will condition the dog to salivate, a conditioned response, upon hearing a bell. This conditioning can be used to explain and treat learned anxiety, helplessness, phobias, obsessive-compulsive disorder, somatoform disorders and sexual disorders.

Operant Conditioning

Operant behavior (eating or dieting/exercise) is activity that is strengthened or weakened by its consequences (weight gain or loss). Operant behavior is influenced by a reinforcement (something that increases the probability of the response). The reinforcement meets a need and is goal directed. **Positive reinforcement** (reward) strengthens a behavior; as well as removal of as in **negative reinforcement**. **Punishment** suppresses, but does not eliminate a behavior. These behavioral principles can be applied in many clinical situations.

Modeling and Observational Learning

A person can imitate or learn through another's performance. Observing the behavior of another can influence a person to behave similarly, especially when the model is rewarded for his/her behavior.

Cognitive Therapy

Cognition is the act or process of knowing. This form of therapy corrects distorted thinking and its underlying faulty assumptions, beliefs, and attitudes. Cognitive therapy proposes that it is not the events themselves that cause anxiety and maladaptive responses but rather people's expectations, appraisals and interpretation of these events. Cognitive therapists believe that maladaptive responses arise from cognitive distortions. Such distortions might include errors of logic, mistakes in reasoning, or individualized views of the world that do not reflect reality.

Family Therapy

Overview

Family therapy is broadly defined as "the attempt to modify the relationships in a family to achieve harmony". A basic assumption of family therapy is that there are certain human behavior patterns that can help people grow and live creatively, while there are others that lead to dysfunction and non-communicative action and result in emotional illness in the family.

In family therapy, the family is viewed as a system in which members are interdependent, a change in one part (member) of the system affects or creates change in all the other parts (members). The focus is not on an individual identified client but rather on the family as a whole. The basic concept of this form of treatment is that it is more logical, faster, more satisfactory and more economical to treat all members of a system of relationships than to concentrate on the person who is supposed to be in need of treatment.

Characteristics of Dysfunctional Families

Families who experience emotional difficulties usually have communication problems. They may discount or ignore each other's communication. They may "scapegoat" one of their members by viewing and treating that member as though he or she is the cause of all the family's problems. They may create "triangles" in which two family members form an alliance and exclude the third person. Passive-aggressive behavior is common.

Family Centered Approach

Family therapy is therapy for the entire family. It is based on the beliefs that the behaviors of one person in the family affects everyone else in the family, and that the presence of symptoms such as depression or anger in one family member is a sign of disorder, pain or problems in the whole family systems. The behavior of an individual cannot be understood without understanding the behavior of other family members. Interventions are directed at the family as a whole and their behaviors, not at an identified client. Family therapy promotes family cohesion.

Technology for Family Therapy

➤ Genogram: A three generational map of family structure and relationships which may be used to diagnose and understand family's history, problems, roles and values.
➤ Communication techniques include:
  – Discussing painful events or family problems openly
  – Clarifying members thoughts, feelings and messages
  – Dealing with anger openly and nonjudgmentally
  – Connecting feelings and facts, never blaming
  – Expressing empathy with family members
  – Experiential and homework activities, such as planning a family vacation, doing a fun activity together or eating meals together.

INDIVIDUAL PSYCHOTHERAPY

Overview

Psychotherapy is the use of techniques that facilitate or allow people to modify their feelings attitudes and behaviors. Individual psychotherapy focuses on the needs and problems of the client. In therapy, two people come together in an encounter that is specifically designed for the purposes of relieving emotional pain, treating mental illness and facilitating change and growth. In a therapy situation, one person is designated as the therapist (the facilitating or helping person) and the other is called client (the person seeking help). As individual psychotherapy develops the client and therapist will discuss some historical information, current challenges, past successes, feelings, needs, and goals. Because of their objectivity and specialized knowledge, therapists generally can be more effective than family or friends in facilitating the client's with challenges and growth.

Levels of Individual Therapy

Supportive

The client is provided a caring, safe relationship in which to explore problems and make decisions. The therapist reinforces client's existing coping skills and does not attempt to teach him/her new coping methods.

Re-educative

The client explores new ways to perceive and behave through a systematic approach. The client and therapist sign a contract that identifies goals and desired changes in behaviors and feelings. An effective approach is reality based focused on solutions and directly deals with concrete issues. Examples include cognitive restructuring and behavior modification.

Reconstructive

The client may spend two to five years exploring all aspects of his/her life through analysis or deep psychotherapy. Outcomes include self-understanding and understanding of others greater emotional freedom, maximizing one's potential, and a greater capacity for love and work.

GROUP THERAPY

Overview

The goal of group therapy is to help individuals develop more functional and satisfying relationships. When an individual's dysfunctional pattern is demonstrated in the group, the task of the group is to assist members to understand the patterns of interacting within the group and to help clients generalize this information to their lives outside the group.

Types of Group

1. *Task groups*—a group formed to accomplish a specific outcome.
2. *Teaching groups*—focus is to convey knowledge and information to a number of individuals.
3. *Supportive/therapeutic groups*—the concern of these groups is to prevent possible future upsets by educating the participants in effective ways of dealing with emotional stress arising from situational or developmental crises.
4. *Self help groups*—composed of individuals with a similar problem.

Physical Conditions that Influence Group Dynamics

Seating: It is best when there is no barrier between the members. For example, a circle of chairs is better than chairs set around a table.

Size: Seven or eight members provides a favorable climate for optimal group interaction and relationship development.

Membership: Two types of groups exist: Open ended groups (those in which members leave and others join at any time during the existence of the group) and closed ended groups (those in which all members join at the time the group is organized and terminated at the end of the designated length of time.

Curative/Therapeutic factors of group therapy (According to Yalom):

- Instillation of hope—client believes he/she will get better through groups therapy.
- Universality—client learns that other group members have similar problems and feelings.
- Imparting of information—client learns didactic information which occurs in a group setting.
- Altruism—client help each other in the group, resulting in increased self-esteem.
- Corrective recapitulation of the primary family group—client's family background influences client behavior and client can relieve and correct early conflicts.
- Development of socializing techniques—client develops social skills in the group.
- Initiative behavior—client identifies with and imitates healthy behavior of group members.
- Interpersonal learning—client's interpersonal distortions are corrected.
- Group cohesiveness—client experiences bonding with the group, group norms are protected and positive client outcomes result.
- Catharsis—group members express feelings, even deep and powerful emotions, and then learn new ways to handle their problems.
- Existential factors—responsibility, existence, awareness and mortality are explored.

RELAXATION THERAPY

Overview

Stress is a part of our everyday lives. It can be positive or negative but it cannot be eliminated keeping stress at a manageable level is a life long process. Relaxation therapy is an effective means of reducing the stress response in some individuals. The degree of anxiety that an individual experiences in response to stress is related to certain predisposing factors, such as characteristics of temperament with which he or she was born, past experiences resulting in learned patterns of responding and existing conditions such as health status, coping strategies and adequate support systems. Various methods of relaxation therapy are presented.

1. **Deep breathing exercises:** Relaxation is accomplished by allowing the lungs to breathe in as much oxygen as possible. Air is breathed in slowly through the nose, held for a few seconds, and then exhaled slowly through the mouth. Breathing exercises have been found to be effective in reducing anxiety, depression, irritability, muscular tension and fatigue. An advantage of this type of exercise is that it can be accomplished anywhere at any time.

2. **Progressive relaxation:** Each muscle group is tensed for 5–7 seconds and then relaxed for 20–30 seconds during which time the individual concentrates on the difference in sensation between two conditions. Excellent results have been observed with this method in the treatment of muscular tension, anxiety, insomnia, depression, fatigue, muscle spasms, neck and back pain, high blood pressure, etc.

Therapeutic Modalities

3. **Modified (or passive) progressive relaxation:** Relaxation is achieved with this method by passively concentrating on the feeling of relaxation within the muscle groups.
4. **Meditation:** The goal of meditation is to gain "mastery over attention". The basic component of meditation include—a quiet environment, a passive attitude, a comfortable position and a word or scene to focus on. It has been used successfully in the treatment of cardiovascular disease, obsessive thinking, anxiety, depression.
5. **Mental imagery:** This method of relaxation employs the imagination in an effort to reduce the body's response to stress. The individual follows his or her imagination in selecting an environment considered to be relaxing, and then concentrates on this relaxing image in an effort to achieve relaxation. Some might select a scene at the seashore, a mountain atmosphere or floating through the air in a white fluffy cloud. Soft, background music enhances the effect.
6. **Biofeedback:** Biofeedback uses a machine to reduce anxiety and modify behavioral responses. Small electrodes connected to the biofeedback equipment are attached to the patient's forehead. Brain waves, muscle tension, body temperature, heart rate and blood pressure can be monitored for small changes. These changes are communicated to the patient by auditory and visual means. The more relaxed the patient becomes, the more pleasant are the sounds and sights presented. These pleasant sights and sounds stops when the patient stops relaxing and they resume when the patient reachieves the relaxed state. It has been used successfully in treating hypertension, migraine headaches, muscle spasms/pain, anxiety, phobias, stuttering and teeth grinding.
7. **Physical exercise:** Physical exertion provides a natural outlet for the tension produced by the body. Following exercise, physiological equilibrium is restored resulting in a feeling of relaxation and revitalization. It helps in strengthening cardiovascular system, prevent obesity, relieve muscular tension, prevent muscle spasms, reduce anxiety and depressions.

ASSIGNMENT 16: PSYCHOSOCIAL THERAPIES

1. Discuss any one psychosocial therapy which you could apply on your patient or one which you observed/assisted during your posting.
   or
   Conduct a psychosocial therapy on a ward situation give by your supervisor.

_____
_____
_____
_____
_____
_____

7
Psychiatric OPD

ASSIGNMENT 17: HISTORY TAKING

IDENTIFICATION DATA

Name: _____ Ward: _____

Age: _____ Bed no.: _____

Sex: _____ CR no.: _____

Father/husband name: _____ Date of admission: _____

Marital status: _____

Number and ages of children/siblings: _____

Spouse/parents age: _____

Living arrangements: _____

Occupation: _____

Education: _____

Religion: _____ Nationality: _____

Mother tongue: _____

Address: _____

Brought by/informant: _____

Diagnosis/provisional diagnosis: _____

CHIEF COMPLAINTS: _____

_____

_____

_____

HISTORY OF PRESENT ILLNESS:

PERSONAL HISTORY:

Infancy:

Childhood: _____

_____

_____

_____

_____

_____

Adolescence: _____

_____

_____

_____

_____

_____

_____

_____

Adulthood: _____

_____

_____

_____

_____

_____

_____

_____

_____

MEDICAL HISTORY:

_____

_____

_____

_____

_____

_____

FAMILY HISTORY:

GENOGRAM:

PAST PSYCHIATRIC HISTORY:

PREMORBID PERSONALITY:

ANY OTHER SPECIAL POINT:

_____
_____
_____
_____
_____
_____
_____
_____
_____
_____
_____
_____
_____
_____

ASSIGNMENT 18: MENTAL STATUS EXAMINATION

1. Identification data

Name: _____   Ward: _____

Age: _____   Bed no.: _____

Sex: _____   CR no.: _____

Father/husband name: _____   Date of admission: _____

Marital status: _____

Number and ages of children/siblings: _____

Spouse/parents age: _____

Living arrangements: _____

Occupation: _____

Education: _____

Religion: _____ Nationality: _____

Mother tongue: _____

Address: _____

Brought by/informant: _____

Diagnosis/provisional diagnosis: _____

2. General description

General appearance _____
_____
_____
_____
_____
_____
_____
_____

Speech _____
_____
_____
_____
_____
_____
_____
_____
_____

Motor behavior _____

Attitude _____

3. Emotional expression

Mood _____

Affect

4. Experiences

Perception

5. Thinking

Thought form

Thought content

6. Sensorium and cognition

Alertness

Orientation

Concentration

Memory _____

Ability to abstract _____

Insight _____

Judgment

Fund of knowledge

7. Any other special point

ASSIGNMENT 19: HEALTH TALK

Deliver a health talk on the topic: _____

Topic: _____

Group: _____

Size of group: _____

Venue: _____

Date: _____

Time: _____

Previous knowledge: _____

Method of teaching: _____

AV Aids: _____

General objectives: _____

Time	Specific Objectives	Content

Psychiatric OPD

Teaching learning activity	AV Aids	Evaluation

Time	Specific objectives	Content

Psychiatric OPD

Teaching learning activity	AV Aids	Evaluation

Time	Specific objectives	Content

Psychiatric OPD

Teaching learning activity	AV Aids	Evaluation

Summary

Bibliography

ASSIGNMENT 20: OUT PATIENT DEPARTMENT (OPD)

Write an observation report of the OPD of psychiatric unit using the following guidelines:

1. Describe the physical set up of the OPD.

2. Mention the various departments and clinics and the services rendered by them.

3. Draw the organizational pattern of the nursing department.

4. Give a brief account of the learning experiences achieved from the OPD posting.

8 Observation Reports

ASSIGNMENT 21: CHILD GUIDANCE CLINIC (CGC)

Write an observation report of child guidance clinic using the following guidelines.
1. Describe the physical set up of the CGC.

2. Mention the various departments and clinics and the services rendered by them.

3. Draw the organizational pattern of the CGC.

4. Give a brief account of the learning experiences achieved from the CGC posting.

ASSIGNMENT 22: DE ADDICTION CENTER

Write an observation report of De Addiction Center using the following guidelines.
1. Describe the physical set up of the DAC.

2. Mention the various departments and clinics and the services rendered by them.

3. Draw the organizational pattern of the DAC.

4. Give a brief account of the learning experiences achieved from the DAC posting.

ASSIGNMENT 23: OCCUPATIONAL THERAPY

Occupational therapy is the use of treatments to develop recover or maintain daily living and work skills of people with a physical, mental or development conditions.

1. Objectives of OT posting.

2. Describe the physical layout of OT department.

3. Give a brief account of the staffing pattern.

4. Activities carried out in the OT

_____

_____

_____

_____

_____

_____

_____

_____

_____

_____

5. Write about any one case that you witnessed during your posting (Brief history of the patient and OT given to him/her).

_____

_____

_____

_____

_____

_____

_____

_____

_____

_____

_____

_____

_____

_____

_____

9 Evaluation of Clinical Performance

Areas of assessment	5	4	3	2	1
1. Clinical skills/technical skills					
2. Planning patient care					
3. Organizing skills					
4. Communication skills (reporting, recording)					
5. Personal qualities (punctuality, honesty)					
6. Appearance (grooming uniform)					
7. Initiativeness					
8. Responsibility					
9. Interpersonal relationships					
10. Problem solving skills					
Total					

KEY

5 — Always knows what has to be done and does efficiently
4 — Frequently knows what to do
3 — Frequently needs to be instructed
2 — Most of the time needs to be told what to do
1 — Always needs to be told what to do

Date _____   Signature of Supervisor

Evaluation   Name of Supervisor

Section 2

IV-Year/VII Semester

1. Community Mental Health Nursing
2. Project Work
3. Ward Administration
4. Evaluation of Clinical Performance

1 | Community Mental Health Nursing

OVERVIEW

The trend in psychiatric care is shifting from that of inpatient hospitalization to a focus of outpatient care within the community. Mental health care within the community targets *primary prevention* (reducing the incidence of mental disorders within the population), *secondary prevention* (reducing the prevalence of psychiatric illness by shortening the course of the illness), and *tertiary prevention* (reducing the residual defects that are associated with severe or chronic mental illness).

Primary Prevention

Primary prevention is defined as reducing the incidence of mental disorders within the population. It targets both individuals and the environment.
1. Assisting individuals to increase their ability to cope effectively with stress.
2. Targeting and diminishing harmful forces (stressors) within the environment (across the lifespan).

ASSIGNMENT 1: PREVENTIVE MEASURES

1. Identify populations at risk for mental illness within the community.

___
___
___
___
___
___
___
___
___

2. Discuss nursing intervention in primay prevention of mental illness within the community.

Community Mental Health Nursing

Secondary Prevention

Secondary prevention is reducing the prevalence of psychiatric illness by shortening the course (duration) of the illness. This is accomplished through early identification of problem and prompt initiation of effective treatment. Nursing in secondary prevention focuses on recognition of symptoms and prevision of, or referral for treatment. The nursing process can be applied in any setting where nursing is practiced.

3. Discuss secondary prevention of mental illness within the community.

Tertiary Prevention

Tertiary prevention is reducing the residual defects that are associated with severe or chronic mental illness. This is accomplished in two ways:
1. Preventing complications of the illness.
2. Promoting rehabilitation.

Nursing in tertiary prevention focuses on helping clients relearn socially appropriate behaviors, so that they may achieve a satisfying role within the community.

4. List the nursing measures that can be administered at the tertiary level of prevention.

ASSIGNMENT 2: HEALTH TALK

Deliver a health talk on the topic: _____

Topic: _____

Group: _____

Size of group: _____

Venue: _____

Date: _____

Time: _____

Previous knowledge: _____

Method of teaching: _____

AV Aids: _____

General objectives: _____

_____

_____

_____

_____

_____

EVALUATION CRITERIA FOR CASE PRESENTATION/HEALTH TALK

1. Teachers personal appearance and movements	
2. Classroom management	
3. Arrangement/organization of subject matter	
4. Presentation	
5. Question-Answer	
6. Use of teaching aids	
7. Use of blackboard	
8. Recapitulation	
9. Assignment/application	
10. Miscellaneous	
Marks obtained	

Time	Specific Objectives	Content

Teaching learning activity	AV Aids	Evaluation

Time	Specific objectives	Content

Teaching learning activity	AV Aids	Evaluation

Time	Specific objectives	Content

Teaching learning activity	AV Aids	Evaluation

Summary

Bibliography

ASSIGNMENT 3: OBSERVATION REPORT ON FIELD VISIT TO A MENTAL HEALTH AGENCY

FIELD VISIT REPORT

Write an observation report of the mental health agency you visited, using the following guidelines.

Name of mental health agency : _____

Date of visit : _____

1. Where is this institute located ?

_____
_____
_____
_____
_____
_____

2. When, where and how did this institute originate?

_____
_____
_____
_____
_____
_____
_____
_____

3. List down the objectives of this institute?

_____
_____
_____
_____
_____
_____
_____

4. What are the functions of the institute?

5. What are the services provided by the institute?

6. Mention the various departments existing in the institute.

7. Draw its organizational structure.

8. Mention the other departments/centers run at the institute.

9. Briefly describe about the physical set up.

10. Draw the organizational pattern of nursing department.

11. What is the staffing pattern and duty timings for the nurses at this institute?

12. Give a brief account of learning experience achieved from this visit.

2. Project Work

ASSIGNMENT 4: GROUP PROJECT

Conduct a group project—quiz, exhibition, seminar panel discussion, workshop.
Write a lesson plan on the topic assigned to you.

Topic _____

Project method _____

Group _____

Size of group _____

Date _____ Time _____ Venue _____

Previous knowledge _____

Method of teaching _____

AV Aids _____

General objectives _____

_____
_____
_____
_____
_____
_____
_____
_____

Time	Specific objectives	Content

Teaching learning activity	AV Aids	Evaluation

Time	Specific objectives	Content

Teaching learning activity	AV Aids	Evaluation

Time	Specific objectives	Content

Teaching learning activity	AV Aids	Evaluation

Summary

Bibliography

3 Ward Administration

ASSIGNMENT 5: WARD MANAGEMENT OF A PSYCHIATRIC WARD

Write the responsibilities of a ward sister in management of the psychiatric ward using the following guidelines.

1. Hospital and unit:

2. Maintenance:

3. Catering:

4. Privacy and dignity:

5. Safety procedures for patients:

6. Fire precautions:

7. Outpatient facilities:

8. Safety of the hospital personnel:

9. Rounds:

10. Duty roster:

11. Report writing:

12. Any other:

4 Evaluation of Clinical Performance

Areas of assessment	5	4	3	2	1
Domain I. Professional/ethical practice					
1. Utilize the knowledge of ethical principles and their implications for nursing practice					
2. Implements the philosophi as policies protocols and clinical guidelines of the hospital/facility					
3. Demonstrate knowledge in the identification and prevention of instances of unsafe or unprofessional practice					
4. Demonstrates in practice knowledge of consumer rights, legal rights					
5. Demonstrates and maintain patient confidentiality					
6. Accepts responsibility and accountability for consequence of own actions and omissions					
Domain II. Holistic approaches to care and the integration of knowledge					
Assessment					
1. Implements and utilizes an appropriate assessment framework safely and accurately					
2. Identifies clients needs					
Planning					
3. Establishes priorities of identified health needs					
4. Identifies expected outcomes					
5. Identifies criteria for the evaluation of the expected outcome					
6. Plans for discharge and follow upcare					
Implementation					
7. Delivers nursing care comprehensively					
8. Identifies, creates and maintain or physical, psychosocial and spiritual environment to ensure optimal health					
9. Provides for the comfort needs of the patients					
10. Identifies and maintains sensitivity to the dignity and integrity of patients					
Evaluation					
11. Critically evaluates the effectiveness of nursing care in achieving the planned outcomes					
12. Determines further outcomes and nursing interventions					

	Domain-III Interpersonal relationships					
13.	Critically evaluates the usefulness of communication techniques					
	Domain-IV Organization and management of care					
14.	Contributes to the overall objective of the hospital					
15.	Demonstrates ability to work as a team member					
16.	Selects and utilizes resources effectively and efficiently					
17.	Utilizes methods to demonstrate quality assurance and quality management					
18.	Demonstrates the ability to coordinate care and work with all team members to ensure client care is appropriate effective and consistent					
	Domain V: Personal and professional development					
19.	Contributes to the leaving experiences of colleagues through support, supervision and teaching					
20.	Educates patients/communities to maintain and promote health					

KEY

5 — Always knows what has to be done and does efficiently

4 — Frequently knows what to do

3 — Frequently needs to be instructed

2 — Most of the time needs to be told what to do

1 — Always needs to be told what to do

Date _____   Signature of Supervisor

Evaluation   Name of Supervisor

Bibliography

1. Barbara Schoen Johnson; Psychiatric Mental Health Nursing, 4th Edition, Lippincott, 1977.
2. Lucindra Campbell Finkelman; Mental Health Nursing, RN Edition, ATI, 2006.
3. Annm Wolbert Burgess; Psychiatric Nursing Promoting Health, Appleton, 1997.
4. Sheila Videbeck; Psychiatric Mental Health Nursing, 2001.
5. Townsend M; Psychiatric Mental Health Nursing - Concepts of Care, FA Davis, 4th Edition, 2003.
6. J Kishore; National Health Programmes of India - National policies and legislations related to health, 6th Edition, Century Publications, 2000.
7. Lego Suzanne; The American Handbook of Psychiatric Nursing, JB Lippincott, 1992.
8. VMD Namboodiri; Concise Textbook of Psychiatric, 2nd Edition, 2002.
9. Kaplan and Sadock's Comprehensive Textbook of Psychiatry, 7th Edition, Lippincott Williams and Wilkins, 2000.
10. Stuart, Laraia; Principles and Practice of Psychiatric Nursing; Elsevier, 8th Edition, 2005.
11. BT Basavanthappa; Nursing Education, Jaypee Brother Medical Publishers (P) Ltd. 2003.
12. SP Agarwal; Mental Health - An Indian Perspective 1946–2003; Elsevier, 2004.
13. R. Sreevani; A Guide to Mental Health and Psychiatric Nursing. Jaypee Brothers Medical Publishers (P) Ltd.
14. Niraj Ahuja; A Short Textbook of Psychiatry. Jaypee Brothers Medical Publishers (P) Ltd.

APPENDIX 1

Nursing Diagnoses in Psychiatric Mental Health Nursing

Box A1.1: Examples of nursing diagnosis in psychiatric—mental health nursing

- Acute confusion
- Anticipatory grieving
- Anxiety
- Bathing/hygiene self-care deficit
- Decisional conflict
- Deficient diversional activity
- Deficient knowledge
- Delayed growth and development
- Disturbed body image
- Disturbed sleep pattern
- Dressing/grooming self-care deficit
- Dysfunctional grieving
- Fear
- Feeding self-care deficit
- Hopelessness
- Imbalanced nutrition:
  - Less than body requirements
- Impaired adjustment
- Impaired memory
- Impaired parenting
- Impaired social interaction
- Impaired verbal communication
- Ineffective coping
- Ineffective health maintenance
- Ineffective role performance
- Ineffective sexuality patterns
- Interrupted family processes
- Noncompliance
- Post-trauma syndrome
- Powerlessness
- Relocation stress syndrome
- Risk for injury
- Risk for loneliness
- Risk for other-directed violence
- Risk for self-directed violence
- Social isolation
- Spiritual distress
- Toileting self-care deficit

Source: Rebrecca and Shives.

APPENDIX 2
Classification of Mental Disorders

Main categories of disorders in ICD-10

Code	Category
F0	Organic, including symptomatic mental disorders
F1	Mental and behavior disorders due to psychoactive substance use
F2	Schizophrenia, schizotypal and delusional disorders
F3	Mood (affective) disorders
F4	Neurotic, stress-related and somatoform
F5	Behavioral syndromes associated with physiological disturbances and physical factors
F6	Disorder of adult personality and behavior
F7	Mental retardation
F8	Disorders of psychological development
F9	Behavioral and emotional disorders with onset usually occurring in childhood or adolescence

Major categories of conditions according to DSM IV

1.	Disorders usually first diagnosed in infancy, childhood and adolescence
2.	Delirium, dementia and amnestic and other cognitive disorders
3.	Mental disorders due to a general medical condition not elsewhere classified
4.	Substance related disorders
5.	Schizophrenia and other psychotic disorders
6.	Mood disorders
7.	Anxiety disorders
8.	Somatoform disorders
9.	Factitious disorders
10.	Dissociative disorders
11.	Sexual and gender identity disorders
12.	Eating disorders
13.	Sleep disorders
14.	Impulse control disorders not elsewhere classified
15.	Adjustment disorders
16.	Personality disorders
17.	Other conditions that they may be focus of clinical attention

DSM IV comprises 16 major categories and over 300 specific disorders.

APPENDIX 3

CAGE

(A screening test for alcoholism)

The CAGE questionnaire consists of four questions. A positive response to one question in the CAGE questionnaire indicates a potentials problem with alcoholism. Two or more affirmative responses identifies problem drinkers.

1. Have you ever felt you ought to cut down on your drinking (amount)?
2. Have people Annoyed you by criticizing your drinking?
3. Have your ever felt Guilty about your drinking.
4. Have you ever had a drink first thing in the morning to steady your nerves or get rid of a hangover. (Eye opener)?

APPENDIX 4

Suicide Risk Assessment

1. Introduce yourself to the patient. Clarify their identity and explain that you wish to talk to them about their recent attempt to harm themselves.
2. The assessment has 6 main components to it:
3. The history of the current episode of self harm.
    - What precipitated the attempt?
    - Was it planned?
    - What method did they use?
    - Was a suicide note left?
    - Was the patient intoxicated (drugs/alcohol)?
    - Was the patient alone?
    - Were there any precautions against discovery (e.g. waited until house empty)?
    - Did the patient seek help after the attempt or were they found and brought in by someone else?
    - How does the patient feel about the episode now? (regret? do they wish that they had succeeded?)
4. Assess risk factors for suicide.
    - Male sex
    - Age > 45 years
    - Unemployed
    - Divorced, widowed or single
    - Physical illness
    - Psychiatric illness
    - Substance misuse
    - Previous suicide attempts
    - Family history of depression substance misuse or suicide
5. Assess the patients mood, especially noting if they are depressed or angry
6. Will the patient be returning to the same situation, e.g. problems at home?
7. What does the patient think about the future?
8. Ask about current suicide thoughts.
9. Thank the patient for speaking to you.

You should summarise you findings to the examiner stating the patients suicide risk. You should also suggest what to do next e.g. hospitalization outpatient follow-up or GP follow-up.

Reference: OSCE skills e learning

APPENDIX 5

Sample Practical Examination Format

	Contents	1	2	3	4	5	6	Total
	Marks	2	10	10	5	3	20	50
Sl. No.	Roll No.							
	1							
	2							
	3							
	4							
	5							
	6							
	7							
	8							
	9							
	10							

Contents
1. Interaction with the client.
2. Nursing need assessment, implementation and documentation (NSG process, health table recreation therapy, ECT).
3. Interview and recording of — MSF/PR/History taking.
4. Practical record book.
5. Appearance and grooming.
6. Viva:
    a. Principles and concepts of MHN.
    b. Mental Disorders.
    c. Treatment modalities.
    d. Preventive, psychiatry, forensic psychiatry, psychiatric emergencies and crisis intervention.

APPENDIX 6

Sample Viva Questions

SET 1

1. Defense mechanism — sublimation, projection.
2. Basic signs and symptoms principles.
3. Cause of organic brain syndrome.
4. S/S by E. Bleuler.
5. Positron emission tomography (PET), single photon emission computed tomography (SPECT).
6. Define anhedonia, circumstantiality.
7. Mileu therapy.
8. Antipsychotic drugs.
9. National Mental Health Act.
10. Primary prevention of mental disorders.

SET-2

1. Defense mechanism — denial, regression.
2. Phases of nurse-patient relationship (NPR).
3. Depression—triad symptoms.
4. Post-traumatic stress disorder (PTSD)
5. Define—apathy, confabulation.
6. Behavior therapy.
7. Hypertensive crisis.
8. Extra pyramidal symptoms (EPS).
9. National mental health program.
10. Secondary prevention of mental disorder.

SET-3

1. Defense mechanism-repression, compensation.
2. Therapeutic communication techniques.
3. Signs and symptons of mania.

4. Somatoform disorders.
5. Difference between seizure/pseudoseizure.
6. Define—LA belle indifference, perseveration.
7. Antidepresants.
8. Admission of mentally ill patients.
9. Crisis intervention.
10. Attention deficit hyperactivity disorder (ADHD)

SET-4

1. Defense mechanism-selective forgeting, fantasy.
2. Interview.
3. Disorders of perceptions.
4. Substance abuse.
5. Personality disorders.
6. Obsessive comulsive disorder (OCD).
7. Behavior therapy
8. Lithium toxicity.
9. Electroconvulsive therapy (ECT).
10. Psychiatric emergencies.

SET-5

1. Defense mechanism-introjection, identification.
2. Disorder of motor behavior
3. Anxiety disorders.
4. Prevention of suicide.
5. Phobias.
6. Legal issues in psychiatry.
7. Post traumatic stress disorder (PTSD).
8. Aversion therapy.
9. Non-compliance to drugs.
10. Preventive psychiatry